THE PURSUIT OF
ENDURANCE

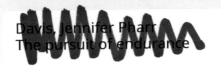

Jennifer Pharr Davis

  DISCARD

THE PURSUIT OF
ENDURANCE

Harnessing the Record-Breaking Power
of Strength and Resilience

VIKING

VIKING

An imprint of Penguin Random House LLC

375 Hudson Street

New York, New York 10014

penguin.com

ISBN 9780735221895 (hardcover)

ISBN 9780735221918 (ebook)

Printed in the United States of America

3 5 7 9 10 8 6 4 2

Set in Arno Pro

Designed by Francesca Belanger

Penguin is committed to publishing works of quality and integrity. In that spirit, we are proud to offer this book to our readers; however, the story, the experiences, and the words are the author's alone.

To Brew

CONTENTS

THE PURSUIT OF
ENDURANCE

CHAPTER ONE

A Wild River Man

"If you can't beat them, you don't have to join them."
—Warren Doyle

I stooped over a thin stream seeping past clumps of dead leaves and earth as thick as coffee grounds. My hands were grasping my shins and my eyes were filled with tears.

I looked up and found myself directly in his shadow. His full beard and round belly absorbed the rare rays of light that penetrated the canopy above us. His presence was unmovable, overbearing yet completely mute.

Why doesn't he say anything?! I thought. *Why won't he try to motivate me or at least place his hand on my shoulder to comfort me? I wouldn't be out here if it weren't for him.*

I'd already hiked the entire Appalachian Trail (AT) twice. But this time it was different. This time, I was trying to become the fastest person—male or female—to travel the 2,189-mile footpath. I was aiming for a fastest known time.

It was day seven and I had already traversed almost three hundred miles of the unforgiving yet alluring terrain. Maine—that dark, full-bodied beauty—had taken more than her fair share out of me. Now, just a few miles into New Hampshire, I was exhausted, filthy, and crippled by shin splints. I longed for a quick, dignified end to the shooting pains, the relentless discomfort.

My current audience wasn't hiking with me. Instead, he had come in by a side trail to check on my progress. I couldn't decide whether I was grateful or angry to see him. I vacillated between crediting him with my progress and blaming him for my near demise. At least his presence gave me a reason to catch my breath.

Through heavy breathing and repressed sobs, I asked him, "How do you know when to quit?"

There was a drawn-out silence. Just when I'd convinced myself he wasn't going to respond, Warren said, "There's a difference between quitting and stopping."

I looked up at his backlit silhouette, then I returned my gaze to the ground. Next to his thrift-store sneakers, he had displayed a selection of vending machine junk food and neon-colored sodas. None of it appealed to me.

Finally, I let out a deep breath filled with congestion and unreleased emotion, picked up a purple vial of synthetic energy elixir—the kind of unregulated ooze they hawk at gas stations—then continued hobbling down the trail. Because we knew that if I stopped, I would be quitting.

I was a week into my record attempt on the Appalachian Trail, and with just one-seventh of the trail behind me I'd already wrestled with the greatest hurt that I had ever felt. The pain from the shin splints was sharp, stabbing, and hot, but the ache of covering nearly fifty miles a day was widespread, dull, and throbbing. It was an all-encompassing agony. I doubted I could make it to the end of the day, let alone the end of the trail. But with Warren by my side, I felt pressure—mostly positive pressure—to keep going. We were two people who shared the same questions.

What was my capacity for endurance? Was it good enough to set a fastest known time? And could I outperform all the men who had come before me?

Because I could still drag one foot in front of the other, I knew that I had not yet found those answers. Warren's watchful eye held me accountable to this very personal and painful scientific query.

A week earlier, I had set off from the summit of Katahdin with a spring in my step. I descended just over five miles on a steep, boulder-strewn path to meet Warren and my husband, Brew, at the base of the mountain. Lots of folks wished me well, or said they believed in me, but these were the only two men willing to drive to the heart of Maine, a place filled with blackflies and bogs, to begin this experiment by my side.

With each road crossing Warren and Brew marked my progress.

"You made it here *this* fast," said Brew.

"You are *this* far behind the record," said Warren.

"You have *this* far to the next road," said Brew.

"You should leave *now* to get there," said Warren.

After hiking 150 miles in three days, our team arrived at the banks of the Kennebec River. Trying to use every minute, I decided to ford the river. Alternatively, I would need to wait one hour to take advantage of a canoe ferry. Steered by a seasonal employee of the Appalachian Trail Conservancy, the canoe ferries afford hikers a safe, mostly dry, transport across the dam-controlled artery.

Warren had crossed the river numerous times on foot, so I followed his sturdy calves into the water. His strong legs moved sideways against the forceful current until they disappeared. Then his waist waded past the white ripples on the surface of the water. Soon he was immersed up to his armpits in the cold, flowing channel.

I kept my eyes on Warren and struggled to keep my toes anchored to the large, smooth stones at my feet. Breathless from fear and the chill of the water, I tried to stay in his wake. My sports bra changed from a light purple to a dark violet as I forged deeper and farther into the river. I listened to Warren as he voiced a steady and concise refrain. "Feet down. Feet down. Feet down." I repeated the chorus in a murmuring echo, hoping to drown out the profanities swimming through my head.

I noticed goose bumps on my skin as my stomach muscles rose above the surface of the water. Soon my thighs slashed through the dark grips of the Kennebec, and after a harrowing and invigorating twenty-minute crossing, I stood dripping wet on the opposite shore. My eyes turned to meet Warren's approving gaze. I smiled and let out a half whimper, half giggle. Warren responded with a deep, bellowing laugh. Then he struck a pose and shouted, "I may have the face of a sixty-one-year-old and the belly of a couch potato, but I've still got the legs of a WILD RIVER MAN!"

Here stood my ferryman: the person who had taught me the difference between stopping and quitting, the man who believed that I could be the first woman to set the overall record on the Appalachian Trail, and the individual who showed me how to keep my feet down and not get swept away by the current.

The year 1973 marked the beginning of the end of the Vietnam War. It was the year of the controversial *Roe* v. *Wade* verdict in the Supreme Court. The Watergate scandal infiltrated the ranks of the White House.

Warren Doyle was twenty-three years old.

He was aware of the civil unrest and he was becoming a proponent of social justice. As a child, he had witnessed his father, a veteran of World War II, struggle to find work and support his family. As an undergrad, Warren spent a summer volunteering in the mountains of Jamaica. Most of the locals there lived in corrugated metal shacks. When his mother came to visit, he refused to stay in the hotel with her. The disparity between the wealth of the tourists and poverty of the natives was so unsettling to Warren that he preferred to spend the night with the homeless street kids rather than sleep on clean white sheets.

The summer after his senior year, he volunteered at a folk school on the edge of the West Virginia coalfields, where he saw the same type of injustice and economic disparity that he had witnessed in Jamaica. Here he met the Appalachian poet and activist Don West, who quickly became an inspiration and mentor.

Warren was the first member of his family to attend college. After receiving his undergraduate degree in elementary education, he accepted a University of Connecticut fellowship that aimed to help schoolteachers understand and implement desegregation through a prestigious doctoral program. He was learning about society and he was learning about education, but he still didn't know who he was.

"I still had questions," he said. "Was I a product of society or was I an individual? I wanted to do something that didn't have an extrinsic reward. I wanted an ultimate challenge—a cleansing."

It isn't uncommon for a young adult to question his identity and the culture in which he lives. But Warren was unlike many of his contemporaries who were drawn to drug-infused music festivals and social protests. As the youngest grad school student in his program, he was an achiever, and he tried to respond to injustice and uncertainty by excelling in his academic field.

After reading of the walkabouts and pilgrimages so important in other cultures, Warren decided that he would hike the Appalachian Trail. But because he didn't like to waste time or money and because he wanted to know how much he could take—and how much he could give—Warren decided to complete the trail in under seventy days.

Warren wasn't always driven. In fact, in middle school, he was a mediocre student; social survival trumped academic achievement. "I was scared to raise my hand in class. I didn't want to stand out. I was afraid if I knew the answers, I would get beat up."

Then one day his fifteen-year-old sister, Colleen, his only sibling, developed a bad headache. Three days later, she died from an undetected brain aneurysm.

"I remember my parents' grief more than my own," said Warren. "I can still see the look on their faces as they came up the stairs to tell me the news. Their expressions were full of suffering. And now they had to put that aside and find a way to try and comfort me, their son, the only child they had left."

When a person is affected deeply by the passing of another, he can choose to die, too. He can turn to self-destructive habits and let his emotions become shriveled and cynical. On the other hand, a grief that deep can also awaken something in a person and motivate him to live life more fully.

"I never wanted to see my parents hurt that much again," said Warren. "I vowed that I would make my life count double."

In May of 1973, Warren's parents drove him south from Connecticut to Springer Mountain, Georgia. Recent heavy rainfall in the Southern Appalachians had caused rivers to flood and roads to wash out. When they stopped on their route to drop a resupply package off at the newly built Nantahala Outdoor Center, the coursing waters of the Nantahala River lapped at the wooden buildings on its banks. In a week's time, Warren would need to pick up his cardboard box filled with several days' worth of rations and replacement gear in order to continue his journey. He left his box of foodstuffs at the outfitter, hoping that his provisions and the building would be there when he arrived.

In north Georgia, the forest service road leading up to the trail's southern terminus was in such poor shape that Warren insisted his parents turn back. Without knowing exactly where he was or how far he had to walk to reach the trailhead, Warren buckled his pack over his blue jeans, slung a two-quart metal canteen over his shoulder, and started hiking.

When Warren reached the top of Springer Mountain, his first thought was for his parents' safety. He doubted their ability to drive down the gravel road without incident. He envisioned the soft shoulder giving way, his parents' car sliding off the side of the mountain.

The first three miles of his hike passed quickly as Warren worried about his folks. But when he arrived at the Three Forks stream crossing, he started to worry about his *own* predicament.

The mountain stream was swollen and the bridge had been washed away. Warren knew he would have to ford the stream, but he didn't want to get his new leather boots wet. When he unlaced his left boot and heaved it into the air, it barely cleared the opposite bank. He then removed his right shoe and threw it with even more oomph, but the added strength caused the boot to hit a low-hanging hemlock branch and drop straight down into the water. The current swiftly carried it downstream.

In a panic, Warren threw off his pack and plunged in, body surfing around boulders and fallen branches until he was able to reach out and grab the nearly submerged boot. With his free hand, he pulled himself up on the bank. Once on terra firma, he dumped the water from his boot and laced it up below his sopping wet blue jeans. After navigating a maze of rhododendron branches upstream, he finally buckled his dry pack onto his dripping body and plodded half shod through the raging waters of the Three Forks to where the other boot was waiting. Warren had exited the mainstream. He put on his shoe and kept walking.

On the second day of his journey, Warren summited Blood Mountain before descending to Highway 19 at Neel Gap, where there was a small roadside store and hiker hostel. He took his boots off, hoping against hope that they would eventually dry out, then he used the pay phone to confirm that his parents were safe.

Less than a week later, Warren found his resupply package right where he'd left it at the Nantahala Outdoor Center. Then he worked his way through Great Smoky Mountains National Park and over the Southern Appalachian high points, Unaka Mountain, Roan Mountain, and Mount Rogers.

Three and a half weeks into his hike, Warren made it to Pearisburg, Virginia. He'd come more than 625 miles. To celebrate his progress, he went straight to the town's Dairy Queen, where he consumed french fries, a cheeseburger, and ice cream. He felt a little queasy, but he ordered a few more menu items for good measure, placing them in his pack before walking back to the trail, where he set up camp.

The next morning Warren woke up, broke camp, and polished off the carton of orange juice, jug of milk, and other treats he'd been saving for breakfast. Hiking out of Pearisburg on Route 460, he started to cross the bridge that spans the New River.

He only made it halfway. He was suspended sixty feet above one of the oldest rivers in the world when his stomach churned and started cramping. He thought about turning back, but it was too late. Maybe he could make it across if he took his time. He took a step. Then he froze. He clenched every muscle in his body, but it didn't matter. There was nothing he could do. Almost a third of the way into his record attempt on the Appalachian Trail, Warren Doyle stood on the shoulder of a bridge in Pearisburg, Virginia, shitting himself.

Warren waddled back to town feeling physically depleted and emotionally ruined. He stopped at the first motel he came to and asked about a room and a shower. When the desk attendant saw him, she immediately called an ambulance. At the hospital, Warren received an IV, and once he started to feel better he called home with an update. When his father heard that Warren was in the hospital, he got in the car and drove south.

Warren Doyle, Sr., a toll collector on the Connecticut Turnpike, made arrangements to take as much time off as possible so he could support his son on the trail. As a parent who'd struggled financially and couldn't put his child through college, this was a very physical way for a father to help his son. With his father's support, Warren got back on the trail and began to make up time and miles. And with his father carrying the majority of his provisions in a station wagon and meeting him at road crossings, Warren could travel farther and more efficiently than before.

It didn't take long, however, for Warren Sr. to learn just how difficult it is to offer support on a long-distance hike—especially to someone you love. Not only was he responsible for having the proper gear and food at hand, but he also had to navigate the unmarked forest roads of rural Appalachia with handheld maps. Even more difficult was the emotional toll of supporting his son.

When Warren hit the mid-Atlantic, the summer temperatures soared and his dad had to watch him suffer through oppressive heat. The triple-digit temperatures and suffocating humidity made it hard to eat and sleep. Warren struggled to balance his electrolytes, but he sweated so much that it was difficult to take in the right amount of fluids and salts.

On one scorching afternoon, Warren came to a road crossing in the Wallkill Valley of New Jersey. His father was waiting for him. As soon as he saw Warren walk out of the forest, he brought out a bag of ice from the cooler in the back of the station wagon. He offered the dripping bag to his son, who was now hunched over in the passenger seat with the door ajar. "Why don't you stop and take a rest? A day off would help you get your energy back."

Without hesitation Warren looked up, and with sweat dripping from his forehead and ice running down the back of his neck, he replied, "Dad, you need to *push* me right now. I need to be *pushed*."

Then he handed his dad the bag of ice, took up his pack, and started hiking away from the car.

The northern latitudes and increasing elevation provided a welcome respite from the oppressive heat. As he climbed Mount Greylock in Massachusetts, he noticed the forest changing temperature and color. The chartreuse leaves of the deciduous trees gave way to dark evergreens and emerald ground moss. He breathed in smells of spruce and fir. His legs felt strong and his feet felt swift.

As he reached the summit late in the day and started his descent into Vermont, he could see the sun setting over the Green Mountains before him. He kept a small transistor radio clipped to his pack, and as he strode gracefully down the dimly lit trail, Beethoven's Fifth Symphony began to play. His gait increased with the music and he started to see how long his foot could stay suspended in the air before touching the ground. It felt like flying.

"I leaped as I had never leaped before. The moment was filled with a vision of hope and the strength of athleticism that comes hand and hand with struggle."

He paused momentarily as he recounted the story, "I remember thinking: Isn't the distance wonderful?"

This was his intrinsic reward. This is what he had come to the wilderness to find. He had obtained an answer and embraced a feeling that was made possible by a grueling journey, one that questioned his makeup and tested his resolve. He knew he could never experience this joy—this nirvana—without suffering through a gut-wrenching, soul-searching inquisition.

After befriending adversity for sixty-six days, Warren reached Baxter State Park, climbed the last mountain—Katahdin—and set the fastest known time on the Appalachian Trail. He left with a greater sense of self and a different perspective on society—an outsider's view.

"After that, there was no going back," he said.

Now he would question everything—and everyone.

I first met Warren in 2004. I was nearly the same age he was when he'd set his record. But back then I didn't know that the Appalachian Trail had records or that Warren had set one. I was just out of college, and despite my having zero backcountry experience, there was an immutable inner voice that said I *had* to hike the Appalachian Trail. In an effort to acquire some last-minute skills before my departure date and to assuage my mother's fears, I enrolled in the Appalachian Trail Institute.

Warren had founded the institute fifteen years earlier in order to help aspiring thru hikers—individuals who hoped to hike the entire trail in a calendar year—accomplish their goal. Since Warren's first thru hike and successful FKT (fastest known time), he had returned to the trail time after time with the goal of completing the entire path. And every attempt had been successful, in spite of the fact that the overall completion rate on the AT hovered just above 25 percent.

It baffled Warren that only one out of four hikers who started the trail would complete their journey. In his mind, the low finishing rate was caused by poor emotional and mental preparation. Most aspiring backpackers spent countless hours sitting behind a computer researching gear, but they neglected to train their brain for the challenge of being in the wilderness—and away from home—for months at a time.

It is easier to debate the merits of a down sleeping bag versus a synthetic sleeping bag than it is to process the reality of shivering all night when the temperature drops below the chosen bag's comfort rating, or to conceptualize the discomfort of the wet and matted stuffing draped over your body after rain leaks into the stuff sack, or to consider the rank smell of sweat and mold that will seep out of the fabric regardless of how many times you wash it. Selecting a sleeping bag is easy; using it for five months is hard.

My first morning at the Appalachian Trail Institute, Warren pulled me aside after the initial classroom session and said, "The AT will change you."

I nodded knowingly but nervously, trying to seem as if I understood the weight of what he was saying.

"Are you really prepared for your entire life to be different? Are your friends and family members going to be okay if you come back from the trail a completely different person?"

To this I had no reply. I opened my mouth but nothing came out.

Having lobbed the grenade, Warren walked away.

What Warren and the Appalachian Trail Institute offered was the chance for hikers to approach the trail with the proper mind-set. Many enrolled looking for encouragement or a pat on the back, but that isn't what Warren offered. Instead, he doled out realistic expectations of long-distance backpacking and he challenged people to consider areas where they might struggle.

If someone was married he asked, "Will you miss your spouse too much to finish?"

If someone had a hiking partner, "What will happen if she quits?"

If someone was on a tight budget, "Are you going to spend too much money at the bars in nearby trail towns?"

Or if someone was out of shape, "Are you willing to lose weight and get fit before starting?"

For the participants who dared to ask, on the last day of the institute Warren would provide them with his calculated probability of their finishing the trail.

I had no desire to ask Warren what he thought the statistical likelihood of my completing the trail might be. Still, he pulled me aside before I left and said, "If this hike goes well then you are the type of person who might consider trying to set a trail record." I offered an uncertain smile, thanked him for his time, and then made a beeline for the door. But I never forgot what Warren said.

Years later I asked him what he meant when he said that I was the type of person who might consider trying to set a trail record. I wanted to know what he saw in me.

"You were athletic," he said. "And I could tell that you had a competitive spirit. That's not to say you were competitive with other people, but you were clearly willing to push yourself. More than anything, though, I could see that you absorbed information well. You were a good student."

As one of his students, I will be the first to admit that I see how Warren has turned people off as an instructor and been the catalyst for turning some people away from the trail. But it is hard to argue with his results. Since the inception of his Appalachian Trail

Institute, of those who complete the course, then set out on a thru hike, 75 percent finish.

Warren's graduates include notable hikers like Bill Irwin, who was the first blind person to traverse the AT, and a man nicknamed "Gutless," who set out on the AT after losing part of his stomach to an aggressive form of cancer.

Warren seemed far more interested in someone's temperament than his or her physical composition—and that included gender. "The trail is still a natural state," he said. "It isn't part of a Western, post-industrial culture that uses strength and religion to oppress women."

He admits that there is an imbalanced gender ratio on the trail and that women contend with greater safety concerns than men, but when it comes to putting one foot in front of the other, he clearly states: "There is no gender bias."

Preparing with Warren provided me with the mental and emotional fortitude to endure early spring snowstorms, rocky terrain, countless mosquitoes, and eight straight days of rain. As an inexperienced hiker and a young woman setting off on my own, I found that his institute gave me confidence and intelligence that I needed to reach Katahdin.

But at the same time, Warren made me look like a complete fool! His methods were so unconventional—and sometimes so unpopular— that most of my fellow hikers thought I was completely unprepared.

Warren does not bring a stove to cook with on the trail. He also does not bring a tent; instead he sets up a Wal-Mart tarp and only if it threatens to rain. He doesn't bury his waste or let camping regulations dictate where he lies down to sleep. He avoids permit fees like the plague and he doesn't filter *any* of his water. Warren's guiding precept is to hike the path as a migrating animal.

Warren's unorthodox methodology stems from his strong individualism and his penchant for questioning authority. However, one can't help but wonder if his departure from accepted trail practices hasn't been influenced by the treatment he's received from the trail com-munity. It is much easier to free yourself from groupthink when the group treats you like an outsider.

Warren wasn't the first person to hike the Appalachian Trail quickly. In 1970, a man named Branley Owen hiked the trail in seventy-three days. But as a result of his youth and his status as a PhD candidate, Warren received far more publicity and attention for his fastest known time. And the response to his feat was not entirely positive. Critics claimed that by hiking the trail in sixty-six days, he hadn't appreciated his surroundings. It must be impossible to enjoy the sights and sounds of the forest, they insisted, if you're hiking that fast. And some feared that by setting a fastest known time Warren was turning a hike into a competition, a trail into a racetrack.

"After the record, I was a pariah," he said. "The Appalachian Mountain Club opposed letting me lead hikes or perform trail main-tenance. They shamed me."

Warren tried to give back. He wanted to champion the trail and assist the trail community. After his record, he offered to help an eighty-eight-year-old trail maintainer blaze a section in his home state of Connecticut. But he was discouraged from volunteering because, as he put it, he had "hiked the trail the wrong way."

Warren wasn't welcomed as part of the local trail club. And in-stead of trying to convince them of the merits of his hike or seek inclusion, he decided to start a hiking group at the University of Con-necticut, where he continued to work toward his doctorate.

In the fall of 1973, he led a series of eight-day hikes. Covering seven to ten miles per day, his group traversed the fifty-six miles of Appala-chian Trail that bisects the northwest corner of Connecticut. That spring, Warren organized a "super hike" in which his coed group of twelve participants covered the same fifty-six miles in a single day.

In 1975, two years after setting his fastest known time, Warren went back to the Appalachian Trail as the leader of a nineteen-person group composed of students from the University of Connecticut.

Together, they hiked the trail in under four months. Nineteen people, four months, 100 percent success rate.

Their completion of the trail as a single unit stirred Warren's hopes and ambitions. He realized that, being an educator, he could provide social and environmental instruction on all things trail-related. Since that first group hike in 1975, Warren has organized nine "expeditions," helping a committed group of individuals to complete the trail as a unit, or as Warren calls it, "an unbroken circle." He has only had one broken circle. In 1977, a woman left the Expedition in *Vermont*, a few hundred miles short of Katahdin. She later finished the trail on her own. Of the 105 individuals who've started the trail with Warren, 104 have finished with him.

How can a man who has increased by threefold his course attendees' chances of finishing the trail, a man who has personally escorted *104* individuals from *Georgia* to *Maine*, continue to be ostracized from the hiking community forty years after completing his first thru hike?

Today, most people who oppose Warren's methods have no idea that he once held the fastest known time on the Appalachian Trail. Instead, they hold a litany of more recent actions against him. For the past four decades, Warren's union with the AT has been as harmonious as his relationship with its governing body has been contentious.

Warren first caused conflict when he spoke out against the federal government's use of eminent domain to obtain land parcels for the Appalachian Trail. Most outdoor enthusiasts were thrilled that the Park Service would want to secure the AT entirely on public land. However, in order to accomplish their goal, the politicians took private land from rural Appalachian farmers. The way Warren saw it, these farmers didn't have much else to hold on to. By commandeering property that had been in a family for five generations, the government wasn't just snatching up their acreage; it was stealing their self-worth and their identity, as well.

Warren is a proponent of working with private landholders to arrange easements, which would allow the trail to cross private property without the government's need to take it. He was also quick to contrast the plight of the poor Southern Appalachian farmer with the deeppocketed owners at Killington Ski Resort in Vermont, who'd just had legislation passed to reroute the trail and run ski slopes across it.

At a time when Baxter State Park dictated that hikers could only summit Katahdin in the warmer months and that they could never do so in the rain, Warren caused controversy by climbing it in the dead of winter as an act of civil disobedience. What part of the wilderness is truly wild if man is not free to make decisions, accept risk, and assume the consequences?

He climbed the mountain illegally in 1977 and again in 1978. During the latter attempt he was arrested and sentenced to pay a twenty-five-dollar fine. Much to the surprise of the judge, Warren chose to spend a day in jail rather than pay.

I never questioned wilderness regulations and fees until I met Warren and, admittedly, I still adhere to *most* policies. But now I wonder about the management and motivation behind the ordinances.

When I hike through Great Smoky Mountains National Park, I am required to pay an overnight camping fee. I am also expected to spend each night at a designated campsite or shelter within the park. But here's where it gets tricky: As an Appalachian Trail thru hiker, I am not supposed to spend the night inside a shelter. Instead, I am instructed to pitch my tent and allow the park's other guests, with preexisting reservations, to set up inside the lean-to. Unless the shelter does not fill, in which case I am forbidden from tent camping and required to lay out my sleeping bag on the wooden boards and with the other campers. If it seems complicated, it is. The regulation is designed to minimize impact, but it creates a confusing and frustrating predicament.

I have spent several cold, rainy hours sitting on the wooden planks of a half-full shelter unable to roll out my sleeping bag in the lean-to and forbidden to set up a tent. There I perch, at the edge of the open-faced shelter, staring into the still, fog-filled forest, and I consider the stories and history hidden in the depths of these mountains. Those are the long hours when Warren's pedagogy takes over and I begin to debate the park's legal authority versus its moral authority.

The Blue Ridge Mountains in North Carolina, Tennessee, and Georgia are the home of the Cherokee. These Native Americans, who refer to themselves in their language as the Kituwah people, arrived in this region around 4000 BC. Their ancestors are buried here and their arrowheads and spear tips can be found in stream beds and underneath heavy ground cover.

Great Smoky Mountains National Park is run by the same federal government that forced the Cherokee out of the Southern Appalachians under the Jackson and Van Buren administrations. The people who once lived here were then made to endure the insufferable Trail of Tears, which ultimately placed the survivors a thousand miles away in the northeast corner of Oklahoma. The small percentage of Cherokee who remain in this region, within the Qualla Boundary, were allowed to stay due to the negotiations of a white man, William Holland Thomas, who had been adopted by the Cherokee but, because he was also white, had the privilege to negotiate to secure private land for his Native American family. Another small band of Cherokee was also permitted to stay in North Carolina, but only after handing over their leader and prophet, Tsali, to a firing squad and agreeing to forgo tribal citizenship and assimilate U.S. culture.

The Cherokee were not the only group that was forced off this land. When the idea for a national park in the Smoky Mountains was broached by a wealthy businessman in Knoxville and funded by John D. Rockefeller, the independent and impoverished Scotch-Irish families who lived and farmed within the proposed park boundary were forced to sell their land and relocate. If they refused to sell, their property was labeled as "condemned" and thus obtained by the government. Many of their former farmhouses and hidden whiskey stills still lie abandoned within the hollows of these mountains. A more physical method was used to displace several small communities in the southwest portion of the park, when the government authorized the Tennessee Valley Authority to build the Fontana Dam to generate electricity for the increased demand caused by World War II. Villages were drowned, families were separated, and a promised road—meant to reconnect the isolated residents—was never built.

Today, the park continues to stir controversy through its infrastructure and designated camping fees. Despite the fact that campers adhere to leave-no-trace policies in the backcountry, the park has marked the land with asphalt highways that intersect the heart of this International Biosphere Reserve and a cylindrical cement tower crowning Clingmans Dome, the highest point in the Smokies—and the tallest mountain along the Appalachian Trail.

To hike there on any trail requires a fair bit of effort and elevation gain, but most visitors drive to the parking lot near the summit and then walk a half-mile paved trail that leads to the top of a viewing platform shaped like a corkscrew. This man-made structure affords 360-degree views from the top of a mountain that is naturally forested.

Is it a victory for accessibility or a visible scar on the so-called "protected" landscape?

I also ponder the positive benefits of the park. Great Smoky Mountains National Park is one of the most visited national parks in the country, an inviting wilderness for the urban areas of the East Coast and a source of pride for the Southeast. The park protects biodiversity, including, for example, thirty different species of salamander. It also promotes engagement, which in turn fosters conservation. Moreover, who am I to judge? I'm white, I'm privileged, and I'm certainly not perfect. My American heritage is as sordid as this park's history. I like hiking here. I'm glad it's a protected natural resource. So does that not make me a stakeholder in the park's sin?

Eventually, I stop fretting over the guilt of the past and simply wonder whether it is late enough in the day to roll out my sleeping bag in the shelter and whether a ranger will stop by the shelter and ask to see my backcountry reservation. When I pull out my paperwork in case I need to prove that I belong at this campsite, I am reminded that this permit and the associated fee were opposed by more than 85 percent of the written submissions during the period of public comment, and disputed by groups such as the Southern Forest Watch, Appalachian Trail Conservancy, and Tennessee House of Representatives. And, once again, I am left processing the man-made stipulations that govern a natural world and contemplating what my personal response should be.

Damn it, Warren!

Warren's greatest feat of endurance is not measured in miles, but in inquiry. He taught me that the pursuit of endurance starts with a single line of questioning. Questions push policies and people to be better. Most often they have easy answers and difficult solutions. But how different the world would look if every individual could cast off the shackles of societal expectation and ask himself or herself, "What am I capable of achieving?"

In the spring of 2015, Warren started the Appalachian Trail in Georgia. At age sixty-five, he was a walking contradiction. His white beard clashed with his youthful eyes, his soft, round stomach opposed his rectangular, rock-solid calves, and his welcoming smile conflicted with his focused gaze. A finish in Maine would mark his eighteenth thru hike of the 2,189-mile footpath. The circumference of the earth is 24,903 miles; Warren had recorded over 36,000 miles between Springer Mountain and Katahdin.

After three and a half months on the trail, Warren had covered just over eighteen hundred miles. He hiked past Lonesome Lake in New Hampshire's White Mountains to a point on the trail that was no more or less special than the long green tunnel that transported him there. And he stopped.

He felt healthy and strong. It was a foregone conclusion that he would finish his trek. But with the end only a few weeks away, Warren realized that he had already accomplished what he had set out to achieve. Emotionally, he had reached his destination and did not feel he needed a physical terminus to complete his journey.

He sat down on a rock beside the trail, startled by the overwhelming realization that he didn't want or need to keep going. His body was not hurting or displeased. The weather was idyllic. It was the middle of the summer in New England, the air was warm, the breeze was cool, and the blackflies had already abated for the season. There were no adverse circumstances affecting his decision. It was with a clear head and a full heart that Warren weighed the pros and cons of concluding his long-term, long-distance commitment.

Warren is a man who expresses his emotion; he will guffaw without an audience and he will sob unabashedly as he passes large groups of Girl Scouts. He does not let social mores repress his feelings, especially when he's outdoors. But after an hour spent sitting and ruminating on that rock, he stood up stoically and started gathering fallen birch branches from the forest floor. Next, he took his collection of twigs and limbs to a nearby sapling, where he started weaving the wood together. He didn't intend to fashion anything in particular, but when he was finished, his creation somewhat resembled a gate.

Most people who walk down the trail will not spot his handiwork. The few who notice it from afar might wonder if it is part of a pagan ritual, a geocache finding, or simply the craftsmanship of a bored hiker. However, if they decide to leave the path and examine the artwork more closely, they will find a small inscription that Warren inked on the birch bark, an ode to Forrest Gump, which reads, "I'm tired. I think I'll go home now."

Warren took the shortest side trail possible to reach the road. And just like that, a journey that started in 1973 with a fastest known time on the Appalachian Trail and totaled over thirty-six thousand miles was brought to an end. He earned the right to stop because he had never quit.

I've known Warren for over a decade, and during that time I have seen him derided on the internet and berated publicly. I myself have strongly—and loudly—opposed some of Warren's views.

Yet to this day I have never heard him swear. The only time I have heard him raise his voice is as a caller, or designator prompter, at his beloved contra dances. And I've never seen him drink or smoke—though once I did watch him devour two pints of ice cream for breakfast and partake of a Chinese buffet a few hours later at lunch.

My husband finds it amusing that Warren has hiked close to forty thousand miles but still has more automobiles in his driveway than anyone else we know. I guess that's what happens when you buy castoff cars for a couple hundred bucks at the Old Dominion Auto-Auction in Bristol, Virginia.

He has detractors, but his independent spirit and his institutional defiance have also earned him praise and a devoted following who label him a folk hero. If you are able to spend some time—and some miles—with him, you realize that the highs and lows are all part of a very human journey.

Forty days after Warren helped me appreciate the difference between quitting and stopping, I once again encountered his imposing and unexpected presence in the forest. I noticed his still-strong body standing reverently in the middle of the Three Forks stream crossing—the same waterway that had swept him and his boot downstream in 1973. The current eddied around his legs as if they were tree trunks growing out of the water. As I drew near, he bent at his waist and dipped his tin cup into the water and handed it to me. I put it to my lips and drank in the sweet, cold refreshment. I was 4.3 miles away from the summit of Springer Mountain and 4.3 miles away from setting the fastest known time on the Appalachian Trail. For the past six and a half weeks, I had grabbed on to the pain and discomfort and tightened my grip. Now it was time to let go.

I thought all my questions would be answered when I arrived at the end. Finally, I could rest—and put to rest the deeply held insecurities and curiosity surrounding my capabilities. Endurance would no longer be an ephemeral concept but a close friend.

I interpreted Warren's appearance at Three Forks as a poetic closure. He was involved in the beginning of my first thru hike and he was waiting for me at the end of the record. But Warren is always more of a prognostication than a period. I should have known that the constant stream of questions would continue.

Once my pain subsided, the fatigue resolved and my calluses eventually fell off. I was left to process what had just taken place. I had established a fastest known time, and yet I still struggled to make sense of it. When reporters, friends, and relatives asked about the record, I hesitated on almost every answer. Even the most straightforward topics triggered rambling, circuitous responses.

Suddenly I had ownership in an emerging sport where even I didn't understand all the rules. People were looking to me to define an underground culture of fastest known times, and I wasn't sure that I could give them an accurate assessment of the endeavor—or my experience on the trail. Demonstrating endurance and understanding it are two separate skills. I could tell people that I set the record, but I couldn't explain why or how I set the mark.

The value of setting a fastest known time is not found in completing a footpath faster than anyone else, but in harnessing the power of resiliency and translating it to life beyond the record. When I reached the end of the trail, I started an exploration of the history, science, and personalities behind the fastest-known-times phenomenon. I wanted to find out what it is that allows someone to continue through insufferable pain and push past staggering odds. I wanted to discover if specific people, personalities, or genders are better suited for the long haul. I wanted to dissect human stamina and discern how we can all find ways go just a little bit farther.

Warren taught me that the pursuit of endurance starts with a single line of questioning. Now, it's time to unearth the answers.

CHAPTER TWO

A Trail of Endurance

"We don't tell them how to enjoy the trail. It's a public resource."
—Brian King, Appalachian Trail Conservancy

"We need places where our feet can connect
with endless dirt and opportunity."
—JPD

Traveling long distances as efficiently as possible has always been a fact of human history, but over the past two thousand years it has shifted from a necessity of survival to a means of travel and communication, a source of cultural and religious significance, and today—depending on whom you ask—an outlet for leisure or competition.

In Australia, the Aboriginal culture sent its sons on a six-month walkabout to signify the transition from boyhood to manhood. This demanding rite of passage required young males to survive on their own while tracing the ancient travel routes, or song-lines, of their ancestors, sometimes traveling a thousand miles or more. When they returned home they were greeted with celebration and trusted with responsibility for the community.

In Peru, there are thousands of miles of pathways that link ancient villages. Many of these pathways predate the Incas. Some, such as the narrow winding paths lining Cotahuasi Canyon, are still used today as pedestrian trade routes. Other trails, such as the Inca Trail to Machu Picchu, the sacred city of the Incas, have become international tourist destinations for adventure travelers.

I went to Peru a few years out of school, and I convinced my former college roommate that she should join me.

"Beach trips are overrated," I said. "Let's catch up on a hike—in

Peru." Sensing her uncertainty, I added, "Don't worry. We'll take it easy on the trail and drink lots of coca tea. We'll be fine."

We threw up more on the trail than we ever had in college.

I still don't know if it was the food, water, altitude, or a combination of all three that put us on an involuntary cleanse, but I recall how poorly I felt as I struggled to ascend the 13,828-foot saddle at the aptly named "Dead Woman's Pass." My memories are clouded by weakness and bathroom breaks, but as I hiked in a hunched-over position I remember the care I took in navigating the loose rocks and steep terrain. It was difficult to find secure foot placement going at the pace of a three-toed Peruvian sloth. I can't imagine trying to run up the trail. But that is how the Incas communicated.

History is filled with the tales of fleet-footed messengers. One of the most well known is the Athenian messenger Pheidippides. The ancient Greek historian Herodotus tells the story of Pheidippides, who ran from Athens to Sparta to seek help in warding off the invading Persian army. When Herodotus refers to Pheidippides he describes him as a *hemerodrome*, which is literally translated as "day runner." He suggests that the *hemerodrome* arrived in Sparta the day after he left Athens, covering approximately 150 miles in less than forty-eight hours. Then, after relaying his plea for help, he turned around and raced back to the battle at Marathon.

The story of Pheidippides has morphed with time and retelling. Nowadays most people believe that he ran between Marathon and Athens, a distance of approximately twenty-five miles, only to drop dead upon arrival. Popular history has shortchanged Pheidippides's ability, but it has also paid him homage by basing the modern-day marathon on his fabled journey to Athens. In the United States alone over half a million people will complete a 26.2-mile race annually.

The research and recounting of early distance feats comes across as male-centric. Back then—as in, in all of history until one hundred years ago—"the pill" was not readily available, and with younger mothers, higher birth rates, and shorter life spans the majority of an average women's life was devoted to childcare. It is logical to deduce that the pregnant nursing mommas were not running through the Andes relaying messages. And if they were, then I really hope there is a petroglyph in some undiscovered cave that depicts the scene.

Delivering infants in the age before epidurals and raising children pre–PBS Kids could be considered more of an endurance feat than running between Sparta and Athens. But when it comes to covering long distances in a short time, there were physical and cultural limitations for most women in history. There is also, however, some evidence that suggests that in many ancient cultures women—particularly preadolescent girls—were an equal part of the pack.

One of the earliest examples of human endurance is persistence hunting. In this tradition, a group of hunters would chase an animal until it fell from exhaustion. It is estimated that the average distance covered in a persistence hunt was nearly twenty miles. The ability to control body temperature, or thermoregulate, allowed hunters to outlast—and eventually overtake—their supper. In modern times, hikers and runners pass many a mile daydreaming about their postrace meal. Persistence hunting takes food incentives to a whole other level.

This method sounds prehistoric, and it is. But in a relatively untouched region of the Kalahari Desert, members of the !Kung tribe practiced persistence hunting successfully into the twentieth century. A female tribe member named Nisa shared memories with American anthropologist Marjorie Shostak of joining her family in tracking and overcoming prey as a young girl. Her firsthand account suggests that this survival technique was more inclusive than previously thought.

For thousands of years distance travel has served to feed one's body and soul. Pedestrian journeys have held spiritual significance— for men and women—in nearly every major religion. One of the five pillars of Islam is a journey to Mecca, known as a hajj. The practice was instituted by the prophet Muhammad in AD 623. Adult Muslims are required to perform a hajj once in their lifetime. Whereas Muslims today use varying modes of transportation to reach Mecca, the original pilgrims walked and traveled in caravans across Africa and Asia Minor to reach Mecca and worship Allah at his holy city.

Buddha identified four holy sites worthy of pilgrimage in northern India and southern Nepal that are commonly visited by both Buddhists and Hindus. A sect of monks living on Mount Hiei, near Kyoto, practices a spiritual discipline known as *kaihogyo*, or circling of the mountain. The tradition started more than a thousand years ago and is still observed by a few devout monks today. The challenge begins with participants walking a twenty-five-mile circuit around Mount Hiei for one hundred consecutive days. Monks who prove their ability in the hundred-day trial then undergo a one-thousand-day walking challenge that culminates with the practitioner traveling more than fifty miles a day for the final hundred days. Historically, each monk would take a rope and a dagger on the trail to end his life rather than quit the sacred journey. This undoubtedly added to his pack weight—and his motivation.

For the past two millennia, followers of Christ have traveled on pilgrimages to the Holy Land and to sites across Europe. The pilgrimage reached the height of its popularity in the Middle Ages, with sojourners crisscrossing Europe to reach shrines, relics, and sites of divine revelation or inspiration. One of the most well-known routes, the Camino de Santiago, stretches its foot-worn fingers deep into France and Portugal to lead religious wanderers to the city of Santiago in northern Spain, where the bones of Jesus' apostle James are believed to be enshrined.

Several years ago, I was asked to guide a high school confirmation class from an Episcopal church on a weeklong trek of the Camino de Santiago. I went into the trip thinking that after successfully leading numerous groups through the backcountry of the Southern Appalachians, taking a handful of teenagers on a wide path through the villages and farms of Galicia should be easy and underwhelming.

But taking a coed group of teenagers to Europe is far more stressful than taking them into the woods. Hormones, readily available alcohol, and a lower legal drinking age led me to walk the halls of our auberges or hostels like a prison guard at night. Although I would describe all of my hikes as spiritual journeys, there was something particularly reverent about taking part in a designated pilgrimage. To follow a route that has revealed divinity to its travelers for more than a thousand years is a humbling, awe-inducing experience. In my experience, backpacking in the wilderness—or trying to set an FKT—allows you to feel free and set apart. Taking part in a pilgrimage gives you a sense of tradition and community. Both are sacred.

Long-distance foot travel has not been considered leisure—or sport—until very recently. In England during the 1800s a form of competitive long-distance walking called pedestrianism arose. It drew such attention that in some instances several hundred or several thousand spectators, even those described as "fashionable females," would come out to observe the participants walk down country roads and cover great distances as quickly as possible. If you think watching baseball is boring, then consider traveling to a dirt road to watch someone walk by! To make it more exciting, betting quickly became interwoven with pedestrianism and both the athlete and gambling spectators had something more to lose than just time.

The most celebrated of these pedestrians was a man known as Captain Barclay. He recorded many walks that are astounding in pace and distance even to the elite runners, speed walkers, and FKT athletes of today. Captain Barclay frequently covered 60 to 75 miles between breakfast and dinner. And, yes, I'm referring to breakfast and dinner on the same day. Once he covered 110 miles on a course boasting ankle-deep mud in nineteen hours. Like Pheidippides, he covered 150 miles in two days, and another time he walked 300 miles in five days. But the walking record he is most well known for is covering 1,000 miles in one thousand hours at the required pace of one mile per hour. It was not the distance or time that made this endeavor so remarkable, but rather the dictate that one mile must be walked each hour for the thousand-hour competition. That's nearly forty-two days of sipping your sleep in minutes, not hours—a month and a half without a REM cycle.

Pedestrianism took off in the United States after it became popular in England. The most celebrated American pedestrian was Edward Weston. In 1861, he walked from Boston to Washington, D.C., to attend Abraham Lincoln's inaugural ball. Traveling a distance of nearly five hundred miles, Weston took ten days to arrive in the capital. Once there, he stayed on his feet and spent the evening dancing. At the time his walk garnered national attention. Today, covering the same distance still earns mainstream media placement, particularly at Daytona or Talladega, where NASCAR drivers can complete the same distance in less than three hours.

Among his other notable feats, Weston averaged more than forty-five miles per day on a walk between Portland, Maine, and Chicago, Illinois. He also walked between New York City and Philadelphia—a distance of one hundred miles—in under twenty-four hours. And he did that when he was sixty-seven. Edward Weston promoted the health benefits of walking and warned the American public of the negative health effects of the automobile. In a cruel twist of fate, Weston was struck by a taxicab at the end of his life and crippled. He died two years later. I always tell people that the most dangerous part of any hike is driving to and from the trailhead. Unfortunately, Edward Weston proved it.

The significance of pedestrianism, pilgrimages, and persistence hunting for modern man, beyond making us modern humans feel like slackers, is the knowledge that the skills needed to accomplish these feats is woven into our DNA. Despite our sedentary lifestyle and rising obesity rates, we are creatures of endurance. It's in there somewhere. We just have to find it—and use it.

Our growing fascination with fastest known times comes with a historical precedent, if not an evolutionary urge, to travel long distances on foot as efficiently as possible. We have been running and hiking through the mountains since the beginning of time. We have spent most of history traveling through nature, and we need places in our asphalt-laced society where our feet can still connect with endless dirt and opportunity.

The Appalachian Trail was never intended to be competitive, but its character has always been inherently challenging. For nearly one hundred years it has drawn out the best in people. It has allowed—if not forced—individuals to surpass their emotional, mental, and physical limitations. It is a trail for dreamers. But it is also a path filled with doers, and most who develop a long-term relationship with it are a combination of the two.

The storied origins of the Appalachian Trail come when Benton MacKaye supposedly climbed a tree on Stratton Mountain in Vermont and peered at the Green Mountains that stretched out before him. As a forester and philosopher he believed that "America needs her forest and her wild spaces quite as much as her cities and her settled places." There was already a long-distance footpath—the Long Trail—that connected the peaks and people of Vermont. Sitting among the branches and staring at the horizon, Benton started to consider the possibility of extending that trail along the Appalachian Mountains that spanned the entire length of the eastern United States.

In 1921, seventy-six years before Bill Bryson introduced it to the American mainstream in his best-selling book, *A Walk in the Woods*, the trail came to life when an article by Benton appeared in the *Journal of the American Institute of Architects,* titled "An Appalachian Trail: A Project in Regional Planning." In it he proposed connecting the highest peaks in New England with the highest peaks in the Southeast.

The idea for the footpath had been delivered, but in order to thrive it needed to gain support from hikers and conservationists and gain ground in the mountains. The first designated mile of the AT was built in 1922 at Palisades Interstate Park in New York. It took fifteen more years and countless hours of backbreaking labor for the footpath to come to fruition. This effort was spearheaded by Myron Avery, who rallied volunteers from regional trail clubs to establish, mark, and maintain the trail.

The trail was derived from a dream, built by doers, and overseen by the Appalachian Trail Conference—a nonprofit organization established in 1925. Assistance was provided by government agencies such as the Civilian Conservation Corps and the National Forest Service.

Since its inception, the trail has been a private-public partnership, evidence that American citizens can provide substantial civic resources with bureaucratic support. Arguably more democratic than the Constitution—at least the part that initially extended voting rights to property-owning, white males, this was a trail of, by, and for the people. It was there for everyone and soon its appeal began to spread. In the words of Myron Avery, "It beckons not merely north and south but upward to the body, mind and soul of man."

Technically, the first completed Appalachian Trail hike served to establish the first fastest known time on it. It wasn't a very high bar. Myron completed the entire trail in sections from the early 1920s to 1936 as he worked to blaze and measure the path—a thirteen- to fourteen-year FKT. But to his credit, some of those sections could hardly be considered a "trail" when he traveled them.

In 1937 a continuous ridgeline route existed between Georgia and Maine. But in the beginning, it was the path less traveled. Back then, the trail was often technical and overgrown. In some places it was confusing and poorly marked. Proper navigation was part of the adventure and getting lost wasn't a mistake as much as it was an inevitability. Myron described it as "remote for detachment, narrow for chosen company, winding for leisure, lonely for contemplation."

The busyness and toil that Benton hoped the trail would alleviate are also the qualities that brought it into existence. Myron was a taskmaster whose relentless work ethic allowed him to build and then hike a trail whose genesis was an article in an architecture journal. Some records suggest that his methods and high standards often left people under his watch feeling underappreciated and overworked. Other accounts hail Myron as an inspired leader working side by side with his volunteers, and long after they had retired for the day.

Perhaps unsurprisingly, given his penchant for productivity, Myron was known for being a fast and powerful hiker. He walked from north Georgia to Gatlinburg, Tennessee, for an Appalachian Trail Conference meeting in 1937, and when he arrived, attendees marveled at how quickly he'd hiked there. Myron even maintained the trail quickly, as evidenced by video footage of him hustling down a single track with a surveyor's wheel to gauge trail distance. I've watched those clips and can attest that, even at normal speed, Avery seems stuck in fast-forward. His pace, plus the fact that he is pushing a device akin to a unicycle with a gaggle of men and women stumbling behind him, makes the clip look like a scene from the Three Stooges rather than from an official government archive.

Benton was not known as a fast or focused hiker; he was a man who climbed trees and daydreamed as he stared out at the horizon. He once suggested that the most notable record should not be awarded to the fastest hiker but to the person who takes the longest to complete it. At the time of his death in 1975—thirty-eight years after the trail's completion—he had not yet hiked the entire thing.

Benton MacKaye and Myron Avery—one a dreamer, the other a doer—gave more of themselves to the Appalachian Trail than any other duo in history and the fact that they were frequently and bitterly at odds is testament to the trail's history, one filled with controversy and conflicting personalities.

Shortly after the trail's completion, World War II began. Many of the volunteer trail maintainers and recreational hikers were pulled away from the woods and away from their homes to support the war effort. The trail was neglected and much of it was reabsorbed by its dense forest setting. By the time the war ended, in the fall of 1945, large portions of the trail would require years to rehabilitate.

In 1948, a World War II radio operator named Earl Shaffer gave word that he was going to "walk off the war." He needed to do something—anything—to distance himself from the memory of watching his closest friend die in front of him at Iwo Jima. So he traveled to Georgia and began his journey north on April 4. He ended at Katahdin on August 5, after 124 days, or approximately four months, on the trail.

One hundred twenty-four days would hardly be considered a fastest known time on the Appalachian Trail today, but it is still shorter than the average five to six months it takes most hikers to complete their journey. At the time, Earl Shaffer had done the unthinkable; he had completed the entire Appalachian Trail in one fell swoop. He had found a path to ease the transition between combat and civilian life. Most people thought it would not be possible—or desirable—to cover the two-thousand-plus-mile footpath in a single push. Some praised Shaffer for his accomplishment; others remained skeptical and even doubted his claim. Critics and admirers alike started referring to him as "The Crazy One."

An unintended gift to history and future hikers on the Appalachian Trail is the journal that Shaffer published after his hike, titled *Walking with Spring*. In it, he provides valuable insight for those who would follow in his footsteps:

> My motto is, "Carry as little as possible. But choose that little with care.
>
> "Most people never in all their lives sleep under the open sky, and never realize what they are missing.
>
> "Someone has said that if you don't like the weather in the Appalachians, just wait a while and it will change."

By the end of journey, Shaffer admitted in *Walking with Spring,* "Trail-hiking had become my way of life. Civilization seemed like a sham."

Earl Shaffer would return to the trail two more times, but not before Lochlen Gregory and Owen F. Allen hiked it together in 1960, becoming the first thru hikers to complete the trail in less than one hundred days—ninety-nine, to be exact—establishing a new fastest known time.

Owen Allen kept journal entries from the trip that were later printed in an anthology of accounts and experiences from the trail's first completers, titled *Hiking the Appalachian Trail.* He describes the journey as "a firsthand lesson in why many close friends have parted company under the demands of long distance hiking."

It is a testament to their shared fitness and friendship that they finished together on top of Katahdin in such a short time. Owen writes in *Hiking the Appalachian Trail,* "There is no question that the satisfaction of accomplishing something that few other people have accomplished was one of our underlying motives, and one of our rewards for hiking the Appalachian Trail. For me, it was recreation in the deepest sense."

When it was over and people asked Owen if he would ever undertake a similar journey he replied, "My answer has been and still is a resounding 'yes!'" But he also provided important insight into the sacrifices and demands of FKT endeavors when he outlined his hopes for a future hike, saying, "I would want enough time so that 15 miles a day would be the maximum hike. I would want time to stop at any particularly inviting spot for a while, time to wait over for a break in the weather so I could see the view from a peak that was closed in on my first trip, time to enjoy long evenings in camp." (Or to paraphrase: *I'm glad I did it, but I don't ever want to do it that way again!*)

From the very beginning of fastest known times, a pattern has emerged in which hikers undergo a more traditional slower hike before—or sometimes after—testing their limits with a record. Although hiking for time is different from a traditional backpacking trip, the first record holders did not suppose their journeys to be either more or less worthwhile than a typical multiday endeavor; there was simply the acknowledgment that hiking the trail quickly was different.

Even the very first thru hiker wanted to experience it in a new manner and with an alternative intent after his first traverse. Earl Shaffer returned to the AT in 1965. He started in Maine and completed his journey in Georgia after just ninety-nine days, thereby tying the fastest known time. The journey also made Shaffer the first person to hike the trail in both directions. The difference in hiking styles between his first hike and his ninety-nine-day adventure is illustrated in the stark contrast in his trail journals. The first was characterized by in-depth accounts and lyrical poetry, the second by brevity, nothing more than his miles and a few bullet-point sentences.

Beyond being the first thru hiker on the AT *and* hiking the trail in ninety-nine days, Shaffer completed the trail a third time in 1998 to commemorate the fiftieth anniversary of his first journey. He was seventy-one years old.

It is important to mention people like Earl Shaffer, Owen Allen, and Lochlen Gregory when discussing fastest known times because this is where the sport has its origins. But it is worth noting, too, that almost all of the thru hikers of the 1950s and early 1960s set records in some way or another.

Gene Espy finished his thru hike at Katahdin on September 30, 1951, and is typically regarded as the second person to complete the trail in a calendar year. There are, however, a small number of trail historians who consider Espy's hike to be the first true AT thru hike, since later findings suggest that Shaffer might have taken shortcuts and alternative routes on his first AT traverse. It only took two thru hikes to create one asterisk. A few weeks after Espy finished, another man concluded his thru hike in Georgia, making him the first *southbound* hiker to complete the trail.

In 1952, Mildred Norman, aka "Peace Pilgrim," and her friend Dick Lamb became the fourth and fifth hikers to complete the trail in a calendar year. Peace Pilgrim is the first known *woman* to complete the entire trail as a thru hike. She and her hiking partner were also the first recorded "flip-floppers." They covered part of the trail hiking north from Georgia before "flipping" up to Katahdin and hiking south to the point where they had left the trail. There were several false reports that the hiking partners were husband and wife. It would have been more culturally acceptable if they had been. But Mildred and Dick were not married, and of the two she became the more accomplished hiker. A self-described mystic, Peace Pilgrim used her long-distance walking to promote peace and vegetarianism. And she was committed. The woman went on to walk more than twenty-five thousand miles and recorded no fewer than eight horizontal traverses of the continental United States. Think about that the next time you feel good for participating in a half-day protest march or completing a 5k for a cause.

The first *solo* female to complete the Appalachian Trail was Emma Rowena Gatewood, otherwise known as Grandma Gatewood. Born as one of fifteen children and mother to eleven of her own, Emma spent most of her life tending to the soil and small children on a farm in Ohio. Her upbringing and lifestyle made her resilient. But it was the threats and hard blows she suffered at the hands of her husband that made her realize she could survive damn near anything, including the stigma of divorce in the 1940s. In 1954, she set out to hike the entire Appalachian Trail, but she became severely lost on the third day and upon gaining her bearings, she abandoned her attempt. The following year, she tried again. This time she completed a northbound thru hike at the age of sixty-seven. When she was seventy-two years old, she hiked the trail a second time. By the time she was seventy-five, she had finished the trail again—this time in sections—thus becoming the first person to report three completions of the trail.

Grandma Gatewood received national attention for her hiking, not only because of her gender and age but also because of her minimalist approach. She hiked in Keds sneakers instead of boots, used an army blanket instead of a sleeping bag, a shower curtain rather than a tent, and a denim rucksack in place of a traditional backpack. She also gave the media great sound bites: "Most people today are pantywaist. Exercise is good for you."

I've yet to hear of a thru hike that isn't unique and impressive in some way.

Some hikers, including Warren Doyle, consider the first real Appalachian Trail endurance record to have been the one set in 1970 by Branley Owen, who lowered the mark from ninety-nine days to seventy-three, a standard that would be exceptionally challenging to surpass.

I was delighted when I discovered that Branley Owen was born and raised in Brevard, North Carolina, a small city neighboring my hometown. His childhood memories include creek stompin', fort buildin', coon huntin', and other activities that lost their full pronunciation in our neck of the woods. He credits his uncles with teaching him how to catch trout, trap opossum, and track a "bar," which is Southern Appalachian speak for a bear. A poster boy for our modern-day Bass Pro Shops and a problem child for PETA, Branley says these early experiences were foundational in establishing a lifelong appreciation of nature.

My exposure to the outdoors came from my father and grandfather, who were devout outdoorsmen. On many occasions I remember being fussed at by my father for tangling a fishing line, and I vividly remember my grandfather biting his tongue and mumbling under his breath when I didn't hit a single clay pigeon in several rounds of target practice. As a young girl, I didn't have much interest in capturing or killing an animal, but I learned that that there was something beautiful about moving among them.

Like Branley, my early exposure to the old Cherokee trading paths and the forgotten railroad beds of the logging industry that run like veins through the forests of Southern Appalachia became grafted into my person. We also share the same heroine: Branley first had the idea of hiking the entire Appalachian Trail when he read a newspaper clipping about Grandma Gatewood. Her story inspired him to start planning, but it was several years before he started hiking.

"I planned for about eight years to hike the whole trail, but never seemed to find the time or the money to do it. Finally I told my wife I just couldn't wait any longer, that I had to go. I quit my job, and she went to work."

Let the record show that Branley Owen had a spectacular wife. Or else she really wanted him out of the house!

As a former college athlete and a member of the Green Berets, Branley felt prepared physically for his journey. Once he started, however, he lamented, "I had trained in the wrong way. To be a good hiker you should be long and lean, rather than strong." Like Owen Allen, Branley Owen shared this sentiment and the following reflections in *Hiking the Appalachian Trail*—volume one, which is an anthology of early appalachian trail thru hiker experiences.

He estimated that his pack never exceeded thirty pounds, which qualified as ultralight by the standards of his era. Today, most lightweight hikers—as well as several of the individuals who have surpassed Branley's mark through the years—start with a base weight of less than ten pounds, not including food or water. In other words, Branley carried a three-year-old while his modern-day competition totes a small house pet.

Even more impressive than Branley's mileage or pack weight was his minuscule budget. He says, "I had planned to do the whole trail for a total of $60, in addition to what I had spent for equipment. However, when I was ready to start, I had only $40, so I completed the trip on that amount."

Forty dollars in 1970 is equal to roughly $250 in 2016. Branley would have had to hike quickly indeed on that budget! At times he was offered money, but he never accepted it. He thought that accepting money would spoil the trip for him.

But there was one instance in which Branley *earned* an extra five dollars. When he walked into a general store at the end of a particularly long day, the manager asked him where he had begun hiking that morning. He shared his starting location, but the manager didn't believe that anyone could come that far in a single day. They made a bet, then Branley asked the man to call a small diner where he had eaten breakfast at 5:00 a.m. The waitress on the line confirmed that Branley had eaten country ham and biscuits at her establishment for breakfast that morning. So the man coughed up a five-dollar contribution.

A thin wallet resulted in a much thinner frame for Branley. He started the trip weighing 217 pounds and finished it weighing 177; he lost 39 pounds in seventy-three days. With that type of result, FKTs might be the next fad diet. Branley says, "By the time I reached Virginia I had learned that a loaf of bread and a jar of peanut butter would make 20 sandwiches. These 20 sandwiches would last me three days. I felt that this was about the best source of protein that I could afford." If that sounds repetitive, it was. Branley supplemented his menu with cattail roots, wild greens, and mushrooms he foraged along the trail. These edibles provided additional bulk, fiber, and nutrients but still lacked the calories and protein his body craved.

As much as possible, Branley collected wild food and slept under the stars. He hiked by the light of the moon, and when he had to, he used a flashlight. Although he grew up as a hunter and an outdoorsman, he admits that hiking the trail shifted his perception of animals and the world around him. "The hike changed many of my attitudes about living things. When I was living in a house and saw an ant walk across the floor, my first impulse was to squash it. When I was out in the mountains and saw an ant, I somehow felt that he had a place in the universe the same as I did, and that perhaps man doesn't own the world, after all."

The individual who attempts to set a fastest known time isn't necessarily blazing down the trail. For many record holders, including Branley, the task is more about long hours than a breakneck pace. He wrote, "I am not an exceptionally fast walker. But I do have one advantage: I often feel as strong at the end of the day as I did when I started in the morning, and I can keep going as long as necessary. I can also move out of camp in the morning faster than most people."

As the first person to place the record out of reach of most recreational backpackers, Branley also received the first real round of criticism directed at hikers who attempted to hike the trail in a short time. He didn't get hit as hard as Warren did, but there was still pushback. After his journey was over, Owen reflected, "The record meant everything to me when I started, but by the end of the hike it meant very little. I have been criticized, both in the press and in conversation, for trying to make this record. One lady, writing in a New York newspaper, said that I walked the trail so fast that I didn't see anything. What this lady didn't understand was that I wasn't particularly looking for scenery. I was looking for something inside myself, and I think I found it."

Four decades later, this sentiment is still one of the best explanations and justifications for attempting a fastest known time. Still, Branley Owen admits that internal focus and long days do not prevent one from appreciating one's surroundings.

"I wasn't always rushing," he said. "If I saw something beautiful I sat down and admired it. I don't believe that just because a person takes 200 days to walk the trail he necessarily enjoys it more than I did. I think it depends on the hiker as to what he gets from his hike."

Warren broke Branley Owen's record by seven days in 1973. But, whereas Warren's father met him along the way with food and supplies, Branley Owen hiked the entire trail by himself and without assistance.

For the first time, there needed to be a distinction between someone who hiked the trail *with* outside help and someone who carried a pack and resupplied him- or herself along the way. Initially, these categories were divided into "supported" and "unsupported" hikes. So while Warren held the overall record on the Appalachian Trail and claimed the fastest supported hike, Branley Owen still retained the unsupported title.

In time, an unsupported hike would come to be known as a self-supported hike. Today an unsupported hike on Vermont's Long Trail would mean that a person covers the 272-mile path carrying all the food and gear he needs for the duration of the trail. It is a feat of endurance—and packing. This feat has never been accomplished on the AT, and even for an expert forager like Branley, the majority of the hiking community deems this type of feat on a two-thousand-plus-mile trail impossible. But, again and again, the impossible has become part of the trail's history and legacy.

A supported effort will typically result in a faster, more efficient record, though it also requires more logistical planning, additional funds, and a vehicle, not to mention the sacrifice and devotion of a friend or loved one. For this reason, far more hikers have completed the trail without support than with it. As a testament to Branley and his journey, records indicate that his self-supported mark stood for twenty years, until 1990.

The fact that Warren received support for the majority of his hike made others realize that you didn't have to backpack the Appalachian Trail. The next person to set the fastest known time on the AT was a man named John Avery, and he was not a hiker; he was a runner.

When he reached Katahdin, John had shaved a mere nine hours off the supported record Warren had set. But Warren had no qualms about John's surpassing his mark. In fact he drove to Katahdin, hiked a side trail to Baxter Peak, and waited for him to finish so that he could congratulate him in person and celebrate his success.

"It is wonderful to see a record holder finish. It brought back a lot of wonderful memories. Now, we had a shared experience. Now, I could talk to someone who could relate to what I had been through. We had a bond. I wanted to meet him at Katahdin so I could welcome him into this fraternity."

When Warren decided he would try to surpass Branley's mark, he tracked down his contact information and rang him up.

"I felt obligated to give him a call," said Warren. "I wasn't asking him for advice. I congratulated him on his record and let him know that I was going to try to surpass his mark if possible. Most of all I wanted to let him know that I was going to follow every white blaze. I wasn't going to take any shortcuts. I would be true to the trail and true to his record."

Branley wished Warren good luck.

In turn, when John reached out to Warren in 1978, Warren extended the same kindness and wished him luck on his record attempt.

Without knowing it, Branley, Warren, and John were establishing the etiquette and culture that would define fastest known times; operating within a certain set of guidelines, their actions established a protocol for future FKTs:

1. Records are based on the honor system. Those going after a record should be truthful in all accounts of their hike.
2. Follow every blaze. The person attempting the record must follow the official trail and pass every current trail marker.
3. When attempting a record, it is courtesy to reach out to the current record holder and inform them of one's intent.

This precedent for FKTs was never formalized, but rather understood. The sport is governed by an undercurrent of integrity. Part of the aura of these undertakings is that the expectations were unwritten. There is something romantic and nostalgic about pursuing an amateur sport that is entirely based on the honor system and completely devoid of a purse for the victor. But there are problems with being a romantic, and there are problems with an unwritten rule book. The expectations of both frequently go misunderstood and unmet.

Within the past decade, countless challenges have been made to the original standards of FKTs. The unwritten rules, the questions that arise, and the evolution of the sport's etiquette are left to personal interpretation.

I knew Warren, so I knew that before I set out on a record attempt, I should first reach out to the current record holder and inform him of my intentions. I held the record for four years, and there were a dozen or so contenders who went after my mark, but only one of them reached out to me before he started the trail. The man who made the effort to contact me was the one who surpassed my record.

It is also important to point out that the individuals who did not make an attempt to establish contact were not all jerks. Some of them were, or at least they came across that way when they posted brash statements about their ability and made assumptions about my record online. But what I took to heart was simply part of a larger trend of announcing a record attempt on the internet rather than person to person.

The merits of trail records are debated in the court of public opinion. And it gets snarky quickly. Hikers are known for being minimalists and nature lovers, but we can also be obstinate and outspoken. We are not all as hippielike and peace loving as our trail scent suggests. Imagine trying to win over Warren Doyle in a disagreement. Now imagine trying to win over a campsite or a chat room full of hikers as resolute as Warren—and with contrary opinions. It's difficult, if not impossible, for the jury to reach a consensus. And in the case of FKTs, there's no judge.

The larger organizations that oversee long-distance trails do not authenticate fastest known times, and most of them refuse to recognize trail records. The Appalachian Trail Conservancy, which was originally founded in 1925 as the Appalachian Trail Conference, has been the footpath's primary guardian and safekeeper for almost a century. Its mission is to "preserve and manage the Appalachian Trail," and it neither verifies nor endorses fastest known times. Neither does the National Park Service, which has been providing management, oversight, and limited funding to the Appalachian Trail since its inception and, more formally, since the National Trails Act in 1968.

Brian King has served as part of the Appalachian Trail Conservancy since 1979, filling several roles, including Public Affairs, Publications, and Archives. For nearly forty years—more than one-third of the organization's existence—Brian has been following the hikers, trends, and management issues involving the path. When I asked him about trail records, he confirmed what I already knew: "The Appalachian Trail Conservancy does not authenticate records; we just file the paperwork along with every other hike report that is submitted."

Brian has a rare knowledge and long history with the AT that is almost unrivaled, except perhaps by Warren Doyle. But Warren and Brian are not exactly kindred spirits.

Warren wears a beard, backpack, and hiking shoes and has an uncanny knack for describing the trail turn by turn. Brian wears a suit and glasses, carries a briefcase to work, and is known for the mountains of paperwork on his desk and the landscape of information in his mind. They have both been devoted to the trail for four decades, pitting more than thirty-five thousand miles of trail against more than thirty-five years of administration experience. Like Myron Avery and Benton MacKaye, both men have been integral in advancing the trail. Warren and Brian are the leading record keepers, storytellers, and historians of the AT. They are living archives.

But at times, Warren and Brian have been very much at odds.

Warren has felt that Brian and the ATC have ostracized him because of his record and his alternative hiking style. Brian, likewise, has at times been frustrated with Warren's constant questioning of Conservancy policy and decisions.

Before I met Brian for the first time, I thought he might have something against record holders and against me. However, I immediately established a natural rapport and friendship with him.

"So are trail records a public relations nightmare for the ATC?" I asked.

"The first time I remember any real publicity arising from record attempts was in the 1990s," he said. "Several individuals were going after the record at the same time and we started receiving calls and letters about it. Many of the ATC members had negative feelings about the records and wanted us to do something, but the stance has always been that if these hikers are not hurting the resource or other hikers, they can do what they want to do. In a way it's no different than a birder or a fisherman going out there. We don't tell them how to enjoy the trail. It's a public resource."

"Are there times when fastest known times are good for the trail?"

"There are hikers whose stories can help the ATC's engagement and outreach. But we don't give any special attention or focus to record setters. We have other more important demands on our time. Right now we are working with a quadriplegic man who wants to hike the Georgia section in a customized wheelchair."

"Well, what about Warren?" I asked with a sly smile, knowing that I was teetering on the edge of acceptable questions. "He felt totally disenfranchised after his sixty-six-day hike."

Brian rewarded my prying with a soft chuckle. "I don't have any problem with Warren's record hike. The problem with Warren is that he is provocative for its own sake and he thinks the rules don't apply to him."

I smiled, knowing that Warren would not disagree, and that he might actually take that as a compliment.

Once John Avery surpassed Warren's time, he retained the record for twelve years. Maybe the fact that John ran the trail with full support discouraged other hikers or backpackers from going after the record. The option was still there to go after Branley's self-supported record, but now the fastest overall time was in the hands of a runner. Could someone with limited resources surpass it?

I had heard rumors of a self-supported backpacker named Ward Leonard lowering Avery's mark substantially in the early 1990s. But when I searched for information about him in periodicals or books, I could not find any concrete information or firsthand accounts of his record. It seemed commonly accepted that Ward had brought the mark to 60.5 days, but I couldn't find his personal itinerary or gear list. I couldn't even confidently say in which year he'd set the record. There were conflicting reports and plenty of hearsay, which was often intriguing but not always complimentary. I couldn't locate any substantial information and I couldn't locate Ward.

Half of the FKT athletes I interviewed were exceedingly difficult to contact and even more challenging to pin down for an interview. When you learn to live on the trail without technology for months at a time, it seems less important to publish an email, host a website, or start a social media page. Even the "accessible" ones were out of reach for several months during peak hiking season. And my requests for interviews were often met with hesitation by record setters who expressed frustration at being misrepresented or misunderstood in the past.

I went to Warren to try to get contact information for Ward, but all he could offer were memories:

"Ward was a physical specimen and the most consistent record setter that there has ever been," he said. "The weather conditions and terrain didn't seem to be taken into account during his journey. He hiked nearly the same mileage every single day. I remember one time we crossed paths at Wayah Bald near Franklin, North Carolina, and we were both cutting fresh tracks through about six inches of snow. When we passed each other we were literally following in each other's footsteps, but his strides were so long that I couldn't keep up."

I went to Brian King for help and he was able to provide a mailing address for Ward, but he couldn't guarantee that it was current. I sent Ward the information I had on his records and a pieced-together biographical sketch based on comments from other hikers. When I put my note in the mail I fully expected to receive a "return to sender" stamp. Instead, after a few weeks, I heard back from Ward's sister.

If you want to get in touch with me, you have to go through Brew, so it didn't strike me as odd that Ward's sister was the one who responded to my query. But I was sad—and frankly embarrassed—to hear that much of what I had heard or assumed about her brother was incorrect or unfair.

To help me set the record straight, I received in return eight pages of handwritten notes, from Ward, recounting his ten completions of the Appalachian Trail and his 60.5-day record, which he held for twenty-three years.

Here's what I learned: Ward set the record in 1990. It was his third time to hike the trail. He walked northbound and spent every night except two sleeping out under the stars.

The following year he did not hike the trail any faster, but his accomplishment is no less impressive. He started in Georgia and hiked to Maine in seventy-eight days. Then he went back to Georgia and did it again, taking eight days off his previous time. After finishing on top of Katahdin, he turned around and walked back to Georgia, this time making it in seventy-five days. Ward hiked the entire Appalachian Trail three times in one calendar year. It wasn't an FKT, but it was a record.

"A record hike is a thru hike without all the unnecessary distractions," he said. "There was an excellence about it."

Ward was indeed one of the most consistent hikers ever to walk the trail. He said that weather and terrain did not affect his miles. On the record, he averaged more than thirty-five miles per day. But in general—on his AT hat-trick and additional thru hikes—he decided that hiking just north of thirty miles per day was the best for his body and recovery. So that's what he did, chewing up miles like a black bear in a berry patch day, after day, after day.

He stretched in the morning and evening and ate three meals a day. He never snacked and he didn't cook. "Cooking takes too much time and requires extra water and gear," said Ward. He didn't carry water on the trail unless he planned to camp away from a water source and, like Warren, he didn't take the time to filter his water.

"It was a natural decision for me to never purify water on the AT, to never hang my food bag when I bivvied out, and to not worry about Lyme disease," he said. "These were nonissues for me because they complicated matters and took away the joy of it."

Ward's hikes were characterized by simplicity, discipline, and routine. Within that rhythm and lifestyle he found pleasure. And he discovered an extraordinary talent for long-distance hiking.

Ward's accomplishments remain some of the most underappreciated feats in the pantheon of FKTs. I'm not sure how much undue criticism Ward received as a record setter. What I do know is that there are many stories out there about Ward's prowess. Some are positive and others are negative, a few of them are true and a lot of them are false. But for Ward the rewards of hiking the trail in 60.5 days, and completing the AT three times in a calendar year, have outlasted his FKT and outweighed public perception.

In his own words, "Having held the unsupported record allows me to know in my heart that I am worthy of respect and that no one may rightly treat me as a second-class citizen or disparage my accomplishments."

I hope that someday I have the opportunity to meet Ward. In the meantime, I am submitting his handwritten notes to the Appalachian Trail Museum so that they can have an accurate record of one of the most accomplished hikers to walk the trail.

In 2008, in order to address some of the debate, ill-defined concepts, and a general lack of information surrounding FKTs, a man named Peter Bakwin started a website on which individuals could record and track amateur records on trails throughout the United States. Peter himself was an endurance athlete who set records on the 211-mile John Muir Trail in California and attempted a record on the 500-mile Colorado Trail. Until he began the website, his research and statistics for each trail were kept in a paper file underneath his desk.

Today, www.fastestknowntime.proboards.com is an invaluable resource, a forum for the small community of enthusiasts who follow and attempt trail records. When I asked him why he created the FKT proboards, he said, "I wanted to provide a place where information was available," he said. "I found that the word-of-mouth accounts were often wrong or contrary. I was really interested in what other people were doing on trails across the country and I wanted to provide a place where they could share their stories."

Bakwin has not only provided a place to track the history and progression of FKTs, but also offered a standardized list of guidelines, including definitions of the three categories—supported, self-supported, and unsupported records.

Peter readily admits, "There are plenty of people who don't follow my guidelines. It's not an official website and I'm not trying to be the governing body of FKTs. I don't want to have to verify or arbitrate claims. I just want to maintain some sense of objectivity and provide a site where information and personal experience can be shared."

In the past decade, more and more, FKT athletes and enthusiasts have turned to Peter's proboards. It's an amazing asset for the FKT community and our history. But the integration of trail records and technology has also been met with challenges, resistance, and resentment. It's easy to post about other people's claims, sometimes too easy, and it's simple to make great claims online without contacting individuals in person. Cleaning up the insults and exaggerated claims on any public forum can be a full-time job, and Peter Bakwin does it as a hobby.

Through this process, I've learned that sometimes the only way to get accurate information is to track down a mailing address, talk with someone's sister, and then wait patiently for eight pages of handwritten notes. In my experience, it can be frustrating, but it also feels far more natural to have to wait, communicate, and read handwriting than it does to look on my phone and read an assortment of posts from a variety of characters.

FKTs offer the same sense of labored authenticity. There is no ease or immediate gratification when it comes to trail records.

I find it ironic and exhausting that we must defend someone's desire to explore the limits of endurance in nature. I know from experience—including "hippie" and "homeless" catcalls—that hiking the Appalachian Trail can be viewed as socially irresponsible. Setting a trail record has also been portrayed as socially irresponsible, with an icing of irreverence or insanity.

But if we ever come up with a time machine and transport a persistence hunter and a Greek day-runner into our modern-day society, it won't be hikers and record setters who look out of place. Instead, it will be our sedentary lifestyle and fast-paced society that seem odd. If we transplanted an aboriginal adolescent, medieval pilgrim, and practitioner of pedestrianism into Times Square, my guess is they would run for the hills—and the trail.

Until very recently, moving constantly throughout the day and spending time in nature were the norm. We are fortunate that, in spite of our industrial footprint, we still have paths like AT where we can get away from the screens, machines, and multitasking of modern society and get back to our roots. Long trails provide a place where we can still live and work outdoors, where we can all reclaim our identity as creatures of endurance.

Throughout its existence, the Appalachian Trail has been a path for dreamers and doers, men and women, thru hikers and section hikers and day hikers. It is a path for runners and walkers, casual recreationalists and record setters. It is a path for those who are hurting and looking for healing. It is a trail that exists because Benton MacKaye had a vision and Myron Avery had a relentless work ethic. It has a story that is told by Brian King and a legacy that is carried on by Warren Doyle. It is a line in the dirt that does not divide us but connects us with one another—and our history.

CHAPTER THREE

The Mainstream Masochist

"Lord, thank you for letting this happen. I wish it hadn't.
But, I know I'll learn something."

—David Horton

In chatting with fastest-known-time record holders like Warren I assumed I'd discover a common thread that would explain how individuals can endure incredible distances and indescribable pain to accomplish their goals.

After observing Warren, it seemed that the ability to defy the odds emerges when a person defines himself or herself as an outlier, someone who simultaneously pushes other people's buttons while also pushing his own limits. My mother would say that I fit this mold—when I was a teenager she liked to tell me that I had oppositional defiance disorder.

Perhaps extreme athletes are naturally able to move freely amid the currents of groupthink and embrace going against the flow of not just what is accepted, but what is thought possible.

But then there's David Horton.

While Horton's personality and accomplishments are unique, his lifestyle, along with his social and religious beliefs, are the essence of traditional American values and as mainstream as apple pie. Horton doesn't go against the flow; instead he's chosen to be one of the fastest, most explosive forces floating the current.

Horton is a dedicated Christian and devoted husband to Nancy, his wife of forty-five years. For more than three and a half decades, he has served as a professor of exercise science at Liberty University in Lynchburg, Virginia. And, as a runner, he has covered more than 113,000 miles. That's four and a half trips around the world.

David Horton goes by many names. His students and colleagues know him as Dr. Horton. His family calls him David, and his running community has come up with nicknames ranging from D-Ho, the King, and Horty to his most prominent title, The Runner.

For the past decade I've simply called him Horton, perhaps because my favorite book as a child was *Horton Hatches the Egg* by Dr. Seuss. In this tale a kind elephant named Horton agrees to sit on a nest so he can keep an egg safe and warm while giving the mother bird a respite. But the mom never returns so Horton has to stay on the egg through bad weather and in spite of the mockery of his friends and neighbors. He even sticks with it when hunters approach and trap him. Then they ship him—still on the egg—across the ocean and sell him to a circus.

(Spoiler alert!) When the egg finally hatches, out comes something new—an elephant bird. And in the words of Dr. Seuss, "It should be, it *should* be, it SHOULD be like that. Horton was faithful . . . he meant what he said, and he said what he meant. An elephant's faithful one hundred percent."

I could never call my friend anything but Horton. He is faithful—and full of faith—and, as a professor, he has incubated myriad young minds and bodies.

His popular running class at Liberty has transformed "couch potatoes"—Horton's description for the neophytes—into avid runners. The class runs through the streets of Lynchburg looking for loose change at the intersections. If Horton is trying to convey the satisfaction of a hard-earned dollar, then dodging traffic and running dozens of miles to pinch pennies should do it.

The students run through the mountains that flank the campus—at night and occasionally through torrential downpours. When the group runs on campus, Horton will yell and prod coeds crossing the quad to join them.

During the semester-long classes, a number of Horton's students will sign up for one of the local ultramarathons, typically one of the "entry level" ones that cover either fifty kilometers or fifty miles. A handful of former pupils who stuck around town are winning those races and others up and down the Mid-Atlantic states.

So how do you persuade people who have never run a 5k to sign up for a 50-miler? And once they've signed up, how do you persuade them to keep going when their entire being is screaming at them to stop?

Well, if you're David Horton you persuade them to sign up by telling them it will be fun. And then when they're suffering, you schlep a megaphone into the woods and alternately berate and cajole them so that the pain of continuing is more bearable than the thought of stopping.

I met David Horton for the first time in 2005. I was less than two months into my Appalachian Trail thru hike and I had spent the previous night by myself in a dank, three-sided lean-to.

It had rained all night and, after pulling on my damp, mud-smeared raingear, I started a steep descent toward the Tye River.

After several miles of focusing on my footwork so as not to slip and of listening to the sound of the rain playing Plinko against the forest canopy, I heard a rhythmic shuffle several switchbacks below. I paused to catch a glimpse of the source of the noise and found myself on course for a face-to-face encounter with a tall, middle-aged man who was running. I was struggling to navigate one of the more technical stretches of trail in the southern half of the AT, so it was difficult to fathom a person having the ability or the desire to run up it.

I stepped off the trail so the runner could pass. But he didn't pass. He stopped, pushed one of the seemingly dozens of buttons on his gargantuan wristwatch, then started peppering me with questions.

"How far are you hiking? Are you hiking alone? How old are you? You're brave! Do you ever run? You should run. Where do you live? What are you going to do when you finish the trail? You should come to one of my races." I'd never heard a man ask so many questions without taking a breath. Even when he stayed in one place, he kept on going.

I was a backpacker who'd spent much of her time alone, so questions never bothered me. But at the same time, I was taken aback by the onslaught and had been in my own head space, so there was a lag time to my responses. I answered as best I could with a combination of nods, laughs, and one-word affirmatives.

I couldn't tell if my gibberish was sufficient to him or off-putting. Regardless, he said, "Well, I gotta keep running! I'm training to run the Pacific Crest Trail (PCT) this summer. Remember to look me up after your hike! And come to one of my races! My trail name is The Runner." Then he was off at twice the speed as before I'd slowed him down. He was twenty yards up the trail before I could muster up my longest reply.

"Okay, my trail name's Odyssa. Bye!"

Many individuals traversing the AT choose their nicknames; some wait for a memorable incident to inspire it, and others willingly absorb the suggestions of another hiker or group.

After I'd spent my first four days on the trail vetoing suggestions like Sasquatch, Amazon, and Stretch, which all harkened back to the social awkwardness of being six feet tall in middle school, I finally settled on a female version of Odysseus. I graduated from college as a classics major. Greco-Roman language, culture, arts, and architecture had led me to the Appalachian Trail instead of securing me gainful employment, but I was still proud of my education and I couldn't help but see similarities between Homer's *Odyssey* and the Appalachian Trail.

"The Runner" rang a bell as a trail name, but I knew I hadn't met anyone else on my hike who shared it. Then it hit me . . . "The

Runner." David Horton was the guy who set the fastest known time on the Appalachian Trail in 1991.

Horton's reputation on the trail is bigger than his personality, and that's saying something. In central Virginia, for anyone interested in ultrarunning, the man's accomplishments seem almost palpable when you're on the trail. He didn't invent trail running but, in the Southeast and the Mid-Atlantic, he might as well have. Most of his 113,000 lifetime miles have been logged on the Appalachian Trail near the Blue Ridge Parkway, the forested ridgelines that flank the James River, and the fields and hollows of the Tye River Valley.

Though these mountains are his home, he's garnered victories and accolades across the United States. In his prime, David Horton was arguably the best ultrarunner in the country.

In the 1970s and 1980s, running more than a marathon's distance—and along mountain trails, to boot—was classified as psychosis more than sport. At a time when games like Frogger and Super Mario Brothers were taking off, David Horton started creating his own obstacle course outside, seeing how far and how fast he could go. There weren't many official ultramarathons then, but Horton researched all the endurance events he could find and started traveling the country to take part.

In his career, he won thirty-eight "ultras." Some were prestigious, like the JFK 50-miler, which is the only ultramarathon course permitted to use a portion of the Appalachian Trail. Others were notoriously punishing, like the Hardrock 100-miler, held in the San Juan Mountains of Colorado and boasting over *sixty-seven thousand feet* of elevation change with an average altitude of eleven thousand feet above sea level.

In 2001, David became only the second person, and the first American, to finish the infamous one-hundred-mile Barkley Marathon. Known affectionately as "the race that eats its young," the

Barkley is generally considered to be the hardest ultrarunning event in the world. It is less a race than an emotional gauntlet set amid a physical obstacle course, and there is something similar in the DNA of an FKT athlete and a Barkley finisher. In its thirty-year history, with a remarkably experienced and talented field and a whopping sixty-hour cutoff, there have been only fourteen people to finish the race. Nearly half of those finishers have also held records on American long trails.

As impressive as Horton's accomplishments are, it's his contributions that have earned him recognition as a pioneer and a "godfather" in the ultrarunning community. Back in central Virginia, he founded and directed races and fun runs alike, allowing thousands of others to know what it feels like to run . . . and run . . . and run some more.

It's not an exaggeration to say that David Horton started an ultrarunning revolution. And, of all places, he did in Lynchburg, Virginia, one of the more conservative—and unusual—towns in the country. The town that invented the cigarette-rolling machine and the over-the-counter enema. The town where an ill-fated eugenics experiment led to the sterilization of more than eighty-three hundred individuals at the Virginia State Colony for Epileptics and Feebleminded. The town where controversial televangelist Jerry Falwell lived and founded a thriving evangelical Christian school called Liberty University. Now, thanks to David Horton, Lynchburg has a reputation as being *the* East Coast hub for mountain trails and distance running.

Almost a year to the date after our encounter, I drove to central Virginia to run my first ultramarathon. The Promise Land 50k is held at a youth camp located between the hamlets of Bedford and Big Island.

When I pulled in Friday evening just before dark, I saw a field filled with cars and tents, a campfire and cookout at a nearby pavilion, and dozens of people in synthetic tees and colorful running shoes, scurrying to and fro and looking very, *very* fit.

I felt at home and completely out of place at the same time. The tents and campfires were a welcome sign, but the spandex—so . . . much . . . spandex—made me feel frumpy, not to mention out of shape.

I had not been running much and I hadn't trained for the event, but I *had* been doing day hikes and overnights with a full backpack. I figured if I could backpack 31 miles in ten or twelve hours, I could probably run the same distance a little faster. Truthfully, signing up for my first ultra race was an excuse for a second encounter with The Runner. A few months after I crossed paths with David Horton near the Tye River, he successfully completed the 2,663-mile Pacific Crest Trail in sixty-six days, setting a new fastest known time there. It was incomprehensible to me that someone could cover that distance so quickly. I was planning to head west in a few weeks, and I doubted my ability to cover the same terrain over the course of five months.

I wanted to pick his brain about the PCT, to ask him about the water caches in the desert and if he'd had any trouble with rattlesnakes and scorpions. I wanted to know about snow levels in the High Sierras and what combination of crampons, ice axe, and trekking poles worked best on sun cups and snowfields. I wanted to inquire about navigation and wildfires. In short, I wanted to grill him in the same way that he had grilled me on the trail the year before. I was leaving in less than four weeks and with much still unknown. I needed David Horton's help.

When I met Horton on the Appalachian Trail, I'd had his undivided attention. And when I met him again at the Promise Land 50k, I received the same level of attention—for about two minutes. He made me feel warm and welcome. He got me excited and quelled my nerves about the race. Then, as quickly as he'd continued running on the Appalachian Trail, he left me standing at the registration desk to personally greet another race participant, and then another, then another. My time was up and I hadn't formulated a single question.

I picked up my race packet and headed back to my car. I walked past a picnic table where a few runners were laughing and conversing and I overhead them talking about other, *longer* ultra races. They chatted as if they had been friends for a long time. I kept my head down and walked faster. Any positive energy I'd gained from my quick encounter with Horton had waned and I was once again feeling like an impostor and an outsider.

I opened the trunk of my SUV so I could crawl in, pull a down sleeping bag over my face, and try to catch some shuteye. Before I could get situated, I heard someone say, "Hey, you're Jennifer, right? Horty told me about you. You hiked the AT last year. Do you want a drink?"

The voice came from under a headlamp at the picnic table. I hesitated, surprised that someone at the race would know who I was. I slowly walked over to say hello and take a seat.

Before I knew it an hour and a half had passed. I listened to trail stories and drank a beer. I decided I should probably have just one drink the night before my first ultra. The others drank copiously and seemed a bit more confident in their prerace carbo-loading.

One of the runners at the table also happened to be a hiker. He had thru-hiked the AT back in the early nineties. And I met a female runner who was my age, twenty-two. They looked more like runners than I did, but I had a lot more in common with them than I'd anticipated.

The next morning, I emerged from my car an hour or so before the sun came up. Fifteen minutes later, with the help of a flashlight, I was following large, well-defined calf muscles uphill. I'd read somewhere that it was sound strategy to hike uphill and run the flats and downhills.

As I hiked up this first steep mountain in the dark, I passed dozens of people, even those who were, at least by definition, running. It made me feel good to realize that I could compete with the runners by hiking. As soon as we reached the summit and I started to jog, every one of them raced past me. On the next climb, I caught them again. I was better at hiking. They were better at running. The game of leapfrog continued throughout the morning.

Early on, and despite a downpour that accompanied the daylight, I enjoyed the race. Not having to carry a pack and encountering aid stations every few miles felt like a vacation compared to a thru hike. I felt very light. And my joy at the frequent refreshments did not go unnoticed. After stopping for several minutes at the third aid station to sample peanut butter and jelly sandwiches, pretzels, M&Ms, a handful of Cheez-Its, and some Oreos, I was told by the woman on the other side of the folding table, "It's not a buffet, dear. You need to keep running."

When you thru-hike, it's common for folks to bring food and drinks to road crossings for the hikers. This kindness is known as trail magic. A by-product of this generosity is enjoying the subsequent spectacle: Hikers can consume ghastly quantities of food in a short period. Moving forward, I realized I'd need to differentiate between trail magic and ultrarunning aid stations.

I made it to mile 20 before soreness and fatigue devolved into pain and misery. The hiking was still easy, but my run transitioned to a tired shuffle. I tried to find a second wind, channel my inner runner. I knew she was in there somewhere.

Before I discovered the AT, I'd always considered myself more a runner than a hiker. At the academically rigorous boarding school I'd attended, my release, my therapy, was running.

Every school day, I woke up at 6:00 a.m. and ran three miles around the deserted track. I ran in the rain and the snow, I ran with my eyes half-open from staying up all night to study. I ran with tears rolling down my face after breaking up with a boyfriend. I wanted to run away from my problems. But that can be hard to do on a track.

In college, I ran for fun. I was no longer trying to outrun my problems; instead, running became a form of exploration. I ran in different neighborhoods, forests, and parks. Before Thanksgiving of my freshman year, I completed a half marathon. A month later, I came home for Christmas break and surprised my folks by telling them I'd finished my first full marathon.

Discovering long-distance running was liberating and empowering. It also led me to the Appalachian Trail. If 26.2 miles felt *this* good, I reasoned, 2,000-plus must be *euphoric*.

I learned that endorphins don't last five months.

My Appalachian Trail thru hike was hardly euphoric. And this fifty-kilometer race kept getting worse.

Around mile 27 it started to rain again. Now skin was chafing against my loose running shorts. No wonder everyone else was wearing spandex! My right hip flexors were shot, my quads were screaming, and a thin white film had glued my cracked, chapped lips to the front of my teeth. At the final aid station, I skipped the food altogether and opted instead for Vaseline and ibuprofen. Then I started down the final descent. With every stride I could tell that both of my pointer toes and the big toe on my left foot were bidding good-bye to their toenails.

I heard Horton in the distance announcing the names of runners and greeting them as they neared the finish line. A bullhorn had never sounded so sweet. As soon as I crossed the arbitrary white line in the grass, Horton engulfed me in his arms and supported my weight. My entire body was aching, but I'd made it through the rain, the mountains, and the unknown recesses of my own mind in just seven hours. I was smiling, sweating and hurting, but in Horton's embrace, I knew also that I was an ultrarunner.

Horton gave me one of the best hugs I had ever had. I still remember it. Then the next runner came into view and he greeted him by name and opened his arms yet again.

I staggered away from the finish line and toward my vehicle. My friends from the night before were sitting at the same picnic table, still drinking beer. They barely looked fatigued. Had they even run the race?

Not only had they run the race, but a couple of them had won it. They'd grossly understated their abilities the previous night. The thru hiker was the overall winner and the twenty-two-year-old took first place for females. I was struck by the fact that the top runners at the event had been so welcoming and kind to a complete novice. I also determined that if I wanted to do better at my *next* ultra, I'd need to consume a lot more beer.

As I drove away from Promise Land, my body settled into a sort of "rigor mortis light" that would take a week to undo. I hadn't spent much time with Horton, but he had helped me immensely. My questions had been put to rest, and for the very first time leading up to my West Coast adventure, I felt more capable than self-conscious—prepared to hike the Pacific Crest Trail, even with just seven toenails.

While I'd spent my teenage years running three miles each morning to endure high school, David Horton had spent his early morning hours before high school milking cows and tending to chores on his parents' farm in rural Arkansas.

The town of Marshall, Arkansas, is a map dot on Highway 65 just north of Little Rock. The population has held steady at just north of one thousand. To this day, the residents are mostly farmers and blue-collar workers.

David Horton was born on February 28, 1950, the second child of Ezra and Lois Horton. He has fond memories of growing up in a county with only one traffic light. Although his parents weren't wealthy, David recalls that they were "rich with work ethic."

"The thing I learned more than anything else from my parents," he says, "is how to work hard. They farmed the land and milked the cows by hand. Until age ten, my parents had an outhouse and no running water. And I'm thankful for that."

The first time I stayed with Horton at his home in Lynchburg, I was part of an assembly line of friends and family who stuffed running socks and bib numbers into race packets until midnight. Then, after three hours of sleep on his living room couch, Horton woke me up so I could drive the dark mountain roads with him to double-check that the aid stations and course markers were set for the race that morning.

Over a decade later, even without a race the next day, I still leave Lynchburg with heavy eyelids from staying up too late talking with Horton. On a recent visit, instead of stuffing race packets, Horton and Nancy treated me to a dinner of country fried steak, mashed potatoes, and green beans. After dinner, I settled into a plush brown couch in Horton's basement and listened as he bragged about his grandchildren and shared some of his childhood memories.

I was struck by the joy and nostalgia that accompanied the tales of hardship in Horton's youth. I'd been visiting him for a decade and had memories of lying on this same couch, one ultra race after another, listening to Horton wax eloquent about the pleasure and pain that defined his race. These recollections of yesteryear didn't feel much different.

When his parents couldn't make ends meet on the farm, David's dad went to work on the highway crew driving a grader. His mother finished her career at a shirt factory.

"In a way, life was very tough," he says. "My parents didn't have a lot of money or things. They were very poor, but they were happy. They emphasized that I needed to work and that I needed an education. It was expected that I would graduate college, even though neither of them ever attended college at all."

David not only completed his undergraduate studies, but received his master's in 1973 at the ripe old age of twenty-three. Five years later, he earned his doctorate in exercise science from the University of Arkansas in Fayetteville. During that time, he also started a family, and began running.

When he married Nancy, he was only twenty-one and she was twenty. They'd been together all of eleven months. David said, "I'm glad we got married young."

To which Nancy replied, "I didn't know he was going to become a runner. If I had, I don't think I would have married him."

In college, if Horton was running, it was most likely on a basketball court. "I was good. I wasn't a great shot. But I worked hard. My favorite thing was to draw a charging foul. I liked getting run over."

In college, Horton focused on classes first, then basketball. But when a friend talked him into running a mile in a spring track meet, he finished in 4.59. In his first race, he ran a sub-5-minute mile! At the conference invitational a few weeks later, he lowered his time to 4.34. The following fall, he ran a cross-country race for his college and finished second . . . shortly after finishing basketball practice.

But after showing so much potential as a runner, David was burdened with the pressure and fatigue that come from expectations and overtraining. During one five-mile cross-country race, he walked off the course before reaching the finish line.

"I just quit," he says. "I was overtrained emotionally and I wasn't enjoying it. I went back to playing and coaching basketball. I only ran a little, every now and then."

As the years passed, David had less and less time for extracurriculars. He worked hard in the classroom and he kept one to two jobs throughout college to pay for the University of Central Arkansas' two-hundred-dollars-per-semester tuition.

After marrying in 1971, David and Nancy were eager to start a family. She carried their first child to full term, and baby Brian David was born at the nearby hospital, but he died just a few hours later.

When Horton talks about the loss, he doesn't share much information or emotion. He describes the loss simply and then moves on to recount the happy memory of his second son being born in 1974 and the arrival of a daughter two years after that.

Horton's much better at describing physical pain than emotional hurt.

I can't imagine anything more devastating than not being able to bring your baby home from the hospital. I wondered how Horton really felt about the loss and accepted the fact that I would probably never know.

Horton was working toward his doctorate in Fayetteville when he finally started running again. "I finished my first marathon in 3:23.54. And then I kept running for the next thirty-three years," Horton said. "But the Appalachian Trail was my greatest athletic accomplishment."

David can't recall exactly when the seed for running the entire Appalachian Trail was planted, but it grew just a little every time he went for a training run on it or passed a thru hiker backpacking the trail. He kept thinking, "Why do only hikers get to experience it? I want to see the whole thing and know what it's like to *run* from Georgia to Maine."

After dreaming for years—and finally admitting his hopes to Nancy—he started making plans for an AT traverse in the spring of 1991. At the time, Ward Leonard held the unofficial record at sixty days. David's goal was to finish in fifty-six, but he admitted to himself and others that he didn't know what was possible. He wondered and worried aloud about his abilities when stretched over two thousand miles.

David wasn't the only athlete going after the fastest known time that summer. John Avery had set the record in 1978, and a full twelve years had passed before Ward Leonard bested Avery's time in 1990. It was rare to see a single record attempt in a summer. But in 1991, there were three.

David began his journey from Springer Mountain on May 7. Two days earlier, Scott "Maineak" Grierson from Maine and Joe "Gator" Ballant from Florida started on the same mountain and they, too, shared the goal of completing the trail in fifty-six days. Never before and never since had the FKT on the AT been a literal foot race between three people starting from the same terminus within forty-eight hours of each other.

Horton figured he'd know whether his attempt would be a success or a failure early on in the adventure. "The key," he said, "is your ability to get in shape the first week or two and have your body adapt on the trail," because no matter how hard you train, it's impossible to properly prepare your legs and your mind for a 24/7, two-month adventure.

After six days, Horton doubted his body would be up to the challenge. He came out of the Smokies in a storm. It had rained every day of his hike. Standing water on the trail and perpetually wet socks meant blisters covered his feet. After climbing to the trail's high point at Clingman's Dome, he thought that the long descent out of the park would be a welcome respite. David was ready to let gravity do the work. He wanted to pick up his foot and let it fall effortlessly on the trail in front of him, then do the same with his other foot and mindlessly repeat that cycle. But it was impossible to get into a rhythm. Shuffle, shuffle, step . . . shuffle, shuffle, shuffle, step . . . shuffle, step. Water bars had been integrated into the trail by volunteers to prevent erosion and keep the trail from washing out. The strategically placed wooden logs deterred the drainage—and The Runner.

At first they were merely annoying and slowed his pace. But after a half dozen miles or so, every time Horton took another long, awkward downhill step, he noticed an acute pain in his right shin. A few hours later, it felt as if someone were stabbing his lower left leg with a knife. It was an agony that I would come to know intimately on my FKT. By the time the sun set, David was hobbled by shin splints.

The days that followed were torturous. "From the north end of the Smokies to the Nolichucky River 110 miles away, I didn't know if I was going to make it. Every time I urinated during that stretch, it was a solid stream of blood. That was the worst part of the whole summer."

For the most part, David had constant but ever-changing support as he journeyed north. But during this time of agony and self-doubt, he was by himself. The next two days, there wasn't a vehicle meeting him at the road crossings, and instead of running, he strapped the hurt and hardship—plus a heavy pack—on his back and walked alone.

In addition to the blood in his urine and the shin splints that meant he could barely hobble downhill, his right leg, arms, and fingers became abnormally swollen. The hikers he passed didn't think he would   or should—continue. But he did. "I was suffering," he said. "But I could keep moving so I *had* to keep going."

David expressed the same sentiment I felt when I was at the low point of my record attempt. And it was the same message Warren relayed when he told me there is a difference between quitting and stopping. He wasn't willing to let the excruciating circumstances define him or determine the outcome that summer. If he couldn't get rid of the misery, then he was going to learn how to live with it. Endurance isn't the ability to overcome pain; it is the ability to embrace it with no end in sight.

There is no guarantee that things are ever going to get better, but the trail has taught me that if you continue long enough, they usually do. Eventually, David's legs began to heal and he started to feel better, relatively speaking. But the low points of his journey came as frequently as the valleys and stream crossings on the trail.

When he arrived in Pennsylvania in early June, he struggled to make ground over the rocky terrain. In his book, *A Quest for Adventure*, which he cowrote with Rebekah Trittopoe, David writes, "It is rumored that the locals come out every spring with chisels and files to sharpen each and every rock. I found myself feeling sorry for the hikers who spend three times as long as I did in these rocky sections. It must seem like hell to them." Then again, every hiker Horton passed probably felt sorry for a man who was crazy enough to *run* these rocky sections.

As he left Lehigh Gap near Palmerton, he was forced to place his hands on the hot rocks above and around him. With dirt covering his palms and under his fingernails, pulling himself up toward the ridgeline, David hit an emotional wall. He was frustrated with this section of trail, these modest but gnarly mountains, the heat, the humidity. But most of all, he was frustrated with himself for setting out on this foolish adventure. He was hiking above a defunct zinc-smelting plant that had left the surrounding hillside devoid of vegetation and completely exposed. Midway through his climb up the barren mountainside, when he'd had all he could bear and was on the verge of tears, David Horton sat down on a boulder and he prayed.

"Lord, thank you for the heat, the hills, and the rocks. Thank you for the good days and the bad days, for the shin splints, the quad pain, and everything else. Thank you for all the help you've given me in allowing me to live out my dream."

Then he pressed on.

David was a college professor, but he also worked in and around freight companies for more than thirty years. Liberty University was relatively new when Dr. Horton signed his first contract. Initially the faith-based school didn't have funds to compensate professors the way an established academic institution might. So for thirty years, Horton worked a part-time job transporting crates at a warehouse to supplement his income and provide for his family.

In 1988, three years before his AT record attempt, David was working alone in the warehouse, transferring an imposing tower of crates from a wooden pallet stacked too high to a nearby forklift. As he unloaded one of the enormous boxes at the bottom of the pallet, the whole thing shifted and a huge transformer that hid on top of the pile came crashing down.

Five hundred pounds of metal landed directly on David Horton's left leg. The impact shattered his fibula in two places and separated the end of his tibula.

Realizing that his leg was shattered and that he was trapped and alone, Horton prayed.

"Lord, thank you for letting this happen. I wish it hadn't. But, I know I'll learn something."

At first blush, that sounds like the refrain of a lunatic, a religious saint, or someone who's lived through a remarkable amount of pain and has managed to gain insight and perspective few of us have.

"I'm not sure how long I was pinned under there," he recalls. "It could have been a minute, ten minutes, thirty. I don't know. I just remember thinking the next shift wouldn't arrive for six or seven hours. I realized I had to do something if I wanted to get out."

David grabbed the crate in front of him, snapped a wooden board loose with his bare hands, and used it to lift the transformer off his broken leg. Then he managed to drag himself out from under the weight and crawl from the warehouse to find help.

The next few months saw a whirlwind of surgeries, infection, and setbacks. After the initial operation, the doctor decided that the leg wasn't healing properly so Horton underwent a second procedure, in which the doctor aligned his bones with two screws. A few days later, Horton experienced an intense burning sensation under his cast.

"It was massively painful," said Horton. "And, I thought, 'Man, there has got to be something wrong.' I went to the doctor and when they took the cast off my leg was huge, red, and swollen. The infection was so bad that the doctor sent me straight to the hospital to have the screws removed. So, I went into surgery again, this time to take the hardware out of my leg. The infection I had was called Gram negative. It was very bad. They pumped me full of drugs and talked about a possible amputation. It was really nip and tuck there for a while, whether or not I would keep my leg."

After spending several weeks in the hospital, Horton walked out on both legs. Three months later he started jogging.

Now, three years later, he was in Pennsylvania, slowly, methodically gaining on Maineak. His other competitor, Gator, never made it north of the Mason-Dixon Line.

For the first half of the hike, David's and Maineak's paces had been relatively even. But now, each day David began to go a little farther than his itinerary told him he should. He began to realize he could do the trail in less than fifty-six days. And he also knew he was closing in on Maineak. As a hound dog brays and picks up the pace as the scent of its quarry grows stronger, Horton's legs started churning more easily and his sometimes volatile mood stabilized and improved. Now he wasn't just running; he was *winning*.

David could keep tabs on Maineak's progress by reading his entries in the registers at trailheads and inside shelters. Knowing this, Maineak intentionally started leaving good-natured notes solely for his pursuer. He also started writing incorrect dates and times with each entry to confuse the calculating professor. After fifteen hundred miles an endurance hiker has to do something to keep himself entertained and keep the opposition guessing.

It took twelve states and countless journal entries filled with misinformation before Horton caught Maineak.

Horton was jogging down the trail in the middle of the afternoon when he approached the cabin at Congdon Camp in Vermont and saw two men step outside.

"I just knew," said Horton. "I just knew it was him. When I caught my first glimpse of Maineak, I was confident that he was the person I had been chasing."

"It is difficult to explain my emotions at that moment in time. I'd thought about him daily for fifteen hundred plus miles. I could easily recognize his handwriting from the registers. But I had never seen him face to face. I thought I'd be excited to finally pass him. Really, I was excited to just meet him."

Together, the two hiked and ran to the next road crossing.

"Our conversation was brisk, as was our pace, and I soon felt as though I had known Maineak for years. It also amazed me how fast he could walk and talk. There was not a single moment of silence . . . I think both of us felt like brothers and compatriots in that we had been together, yet separate, chasing the same dream."

David was a runner and Maineak was a hiker. But for the next few days, the two traveled concurrently and took turns exchanging the lead. David would gain on Maineak and pass him, but Maineak's steady pace and long days kept him on the trail long after Horton had stopped for the night, and he got going well before Horton woke the next morning. Their competition could have proved contentious, but instead, their shared experience and their common goal forged a friendship. They compared notes on past miles, discussed the upcoming terrain, and took great delight in sneaking up on the other person and scaring the jogging shorts off him.

After 143 miles of hiking together, alternating positions, and sharing the chore of breaking through hundreds if not thousands of early morning spiderwebs, David passed Maineak at Etna-Hanover Center Road in New Hampshire. He thought he'd see him again the next day, but Maineak's miles lagged and he fell behind.

The two men wouldn't cross paths again until months later at a hiker gathering. When David walked up to Maineak, he had to reintroduce himself—Maineak didn't recognize him without a beard.

After 52 days, 9 hours and 41 minutes, David reached the summit of Katahdin. He surpassed the fastest known time by 8 days, and beat his friend Maineak, who reached the final summit in 55 days.

Even with the euphoria of accomplishing such a monumental goal,

David struggled to muster the energy or stamina to descend Katahdin. A northbound hike does not end at the top of Katahdin; you still have to pick a path and scramble over boulders or slide down loose scree to reach a trailhead—and road—at the base of the mountain.

For fifty-two days David had averaged forty-one miles a day. And he was beat up. He had a six-inch gash on his right arm, a deep puncture wound on his left thigh, and, ahem, severe hemorrhoids that he prayed wouldn't rupture.

"I was tired of being tired," he said.

If feeling haggard at the end of his journey wasn't enough to dissuade David from tackling more multiday, multistate adventures, he still had to face the nightmares and restlessness that haunted him when he got home. For weeks he woke up in panics and cold sweats, dreaming that he was falling behind on his record attempt. "It felt as if I were losing ground and like everything was uphill."

It took months to recover. And Nancy didn't exactly welcome him home with open arms and foot massages.

"There were good times throughout this endeavor, and there were certainly bad times. I don't know which outweighed which," Nancy recalls. "It was a very hard and lonely two months for me. I didn't get married to live alone!"

Four years passed before David left again.

In 1995, he ran across the continental United States. Starting in Rancho Cucamongo, California, and ending in New York City, he covered 2,906 miles in sixty-four days. After speaking with the Hortons, it's unclear whether Nancy gave David her blessing for this adventure or merely tolerated her husband's ambition. One thing's for sure, though: David was drawn to challenges longer and more grueling than typical ultra races of the 50k, 50-mile, 100-mile, or 24-hour variety. The Appalachian Trail revealed an entirely different world to David, one even more rewarding than winning legendary long-distance races.

About every five years since 1991, David has planned something *big*. After the AT and his 1995 run across America, he tackled the Barkley one-hundred-mile run in 2001. A few months after I met him in 2005, he set the FKT on the Pacific Crest Trail. And in 2011, he biked from Canada to Mexico along the Continental Divide.

Since meeting Horton, I have closely followed his adventures and often followed in his footsteps. We have done several of the same long-distance trails and I have run almost all of his ultra races. *Almost.*

He hosts a hundred-kilometer race through the Blue Ridge Mountains of Virginia that starts at midnight the second Saturday in December. It's called Hellgate, and some years a handful of runners will be forced to quit because their eyeballs freeze. (In extreme cold and wind, your cornea can literally freeze.)

I refuse to run Hellgate. I hate being cold and I like being able to see.

When I tell Horton for another consecutive year that I am not registering for his winter run, he responds, "That's right, you're just a girl. You're probably not tough enough."

I can't tell you the number of times I've heard Horton say that to me or other women at his races. Now I smile when I see the horror on the face of a young woman who comes to a race for the first time and overhears his sexist banter. I am sure I wore the same expression when I was first exposed to it. Sometimes, it really is hard to know whether he is kidding. His words often come across as offensive and they always come across as a challenge. That's how he wants it.

Horton is not politically correct. He is willing to offend, insult, and demean. The fact that it is done in good humor does not excuse it, but his intentions are never malicious. As with starting a car, he knows if he pushes the right combination of buttons he might just put someone in motion. I will add that every time I finish one of his races or complete another long trail, Horton is there to offer his congratulations and engulf me with a hug.

"You are one of the toughest *people* I know," he says.

He is always challenging the men and women whom he comes in contact with to do something longer and harder than they've done in the past. It's the same pressure he puts on himself daily. Horton isn't very good at scaling down his enthusiasm or his adventures. It is a defining quality and part of what makes him great. But his addiction to miles has taken a toll on his body and his marriage.

Horton's endurance pursuits have strained his relationship with his wife and caused disagreements that, admirably, David and Nancy have struggled through together. Both Horton and Nancy have been forthcoming about times when they didn't see eye to eye. In fact, they still don't see eye to eye. "I may not agree with his adventures or even understand them," said Nancy. "But at this point, I know it's something he has to do."

In a world of social media where we are constantly portraying our best selves, or an even better version of our best selves, it is both unsettling and encouraging for couples to be honest about their partnership. David and Nancy's marriage is a greater testament to endurance than any of Horton's trail records. And it is their faith in God, more than their faith in each other, that has held their covenant intact. They have learned that sometimes you need to believe in something greater than yourself in order to keep moving forward.

David has also dealt with his share of health concerns and surgeries, inconveniences that have hampered and sometimes sidelined him—but only temporarily.

The first real threat to his mobility took place before he began running as a teenager, before he can even remember. It is a story that his mother likes to tell.

When David was a young child, around four years old, he developed an infection between his hipbone and his leg. The inflammation was so painful and severe that this energetic little boy couldn't summon the ability, or even the desire, to walk for a full two weeks. His mother said that every day she would carry him from the bed to the kitchen so he could eat, then she toted him around the farm while she performed her chores. More than once, as she was holding him in her arms, the future running prodigy and record setter whimpered tearfully, "Will I ever walk again?"

"Yes, baby."

David *would* walk, and play basketball, and take up tennis and golf, too. Then, on a spring day in high school, David started to run.

He ran until age thirty-eight, when the transformer fell on his leg at the freight company. Even then, just seven months after the doctor considered amputating his leg, he would run the Old Dominion 100-miler. And he didn't just finish his first race back; he won it.

He ran until 2010, when a pain in his right leg started to slow him down. The doctor said his meniscus was torn, that it and the articular cartilage in his knee were both worn thin. David had two surgeries in hopes of repairing it, including one total knee replacement. When the doctor told him he needed to dial it back, David balked. Not wanting to quit, he did one of the hardest things he'd ever had to do and made one of the biggest changes of his life: The Runner bought a bike.

In his first six years as a cyclist, Horton has put twenty-five thousand miles on his road and mountain bikes—and counting. He cycles along the Blue Ridge Parkway every weekend during the academic year, and every summer he heads west with his mountain bike in tow. He may not have been running, but you better believe he found a way to keep moving.

He dove into riding with the same passion with which he'd embraced running. That is, right up until December 12, 2012, when he was forced to undergo septuple bypass surgery.

I was shocked when I heard the news. An individual who'd never had a drink in his life, smoked, or done recreational drugs, who'd covered more than 113,000 miles in his lifetime *on foot*, had seven coronary arteries repaired. I didn't realize anyone could have seven bypasses, let alone that such a fit person would require something so drastic.

But David wasn't entirely caught off guard. He knew these conditions were hereditary, and that seven of his mother's siblings had died in their forties due to heart trouble.

When David met with the surgeon, he asked, "Is this because of my family? Is it hereditary?"

His doctor said, "Yes."

"But why," he asked, "do I need *seven*?"

The surgeon looked up from his clipboard at David and said frankly, "Because of what you've done, who you are, and what you're going to do."

The doctor knew his patient well. He knew that the stress David had put his heart through as a runner would help him survive and heal from seven bypasses. He also recognized that after a lifetime of activity, David wouldn't be content to live out a sedentary existence after the operation.

The day of the procedure, David remembers being rolled away from his family on the gurney. "I didn't think I would die," he said, "but I knew it would be okay if I did."

"Have your greatest struggles come on trail or off?" I asked.

"Off," he said.

"Have you ever doubted your faith?"

"No. No, I never have."

It was David and Nancy's faith in God that saw them through the hard times. It was Horton's belief that Jesus wanted him to help people become healthy and get moving that encouraged him to pursue a career in exercise science. And it was his faith that helped him overcome loneliness, agony, and despair during the lowest moments of his life.

In some ways, my faith and Horton's are the same, but in other ways, our faiths are very different. If we were checking boxes, we would both label ourselves as Christians, but unlike Horton, I have doubted, questioned, and wrestled with my faith. That said, I don't think I would have set an FKT if I didn't believe in God. And Horton feels the same.

During the moments when I didn't think I could keep going, times when my body and mind refused to take another step, there was something bigger at play. Maybe it was a miracle or maybe it was all in my head. Either way, sometimes in relationships and trail records, you need to believe in something greater than yourself in order to keep moving forward.

I think most record setters have some sort of transcendent purpose that helps them to keep going. For some it might be a love of nature. Others might seek to raise funds for a sick family member, or to commemorate the life of friend who has died, raise social awareness for a cause, or fight against some injustice. But maybe, maybe that's all just wishful thinking. Maybe the only reason people make these superhuman efforts is, as Nancy Horton suggests, pure unadulterated ego.

She says it with a smile and gentle laughter. Still, I can't help but cringe.

It's like hearing Horton taunt me because of my gender. Does he really mean it? Or is he saying it as a good-natured joke?

Does Nancy really want to say that her husband has been driven by a sense of self-importance?

And what if she's right?

What if my own record-setting effort was based on nothing more than hubris?

Nancy knows her husband better than I do, but here's what I know: I know that when I talk to Warren or Horton about trail records, there is a youthful light that shines in the eyes of these men who are technically senior citizens. I notice the excitement in their voices, the tendency to smile more when we theorize about unexplored ways to improve the mark. I'm living proof of how much they've poured into the lives of other people who share their passion.

Both of them have volunteered their time—not days, but *weeks*—to help me down the trail. They have shared their wisdom and offered their encouragement; housed me, fed me, and shared their lives with me. And they've never asked or expected anything in return.

It would be impossible for me to call these men selfish. Despite their flaws, they love too much and too well. And, despite our differences and disagreements, they have always cared for me. They've given me a lot.

When Horton came to help me on the Appalachian Trail in 2008, he shared with me one of his deepest struggles. I never forgot what he said.

Eight years later, he dredged it up again as we sat in his basement.

"Do you know what I wrestle with the most?" he asked.

Curious if his response would be the same, I looked up and waited for it.

"Insecurity."

David Horton is consistent. The man who has never doubted that there is a God—the devoted husband, the dedicated teacher, one of the best endurance athletes in history—doesn't question others, but he doubts his own self-worth and he always has.

I don't think that's ego or a matter of pride. I think it's something that nearly everyone struggles with, no matter his or her level of confidence or accomplishment. Horton has shown me that you don't have to overcome your insecurity to realize your potential. As with the unending hurt of an FKT, you can strap it on your back, take it with you, and not let it prevent you from pursuing your dreams.

The last time I followed David Horton into the woods, it was a warm, late winter afternoon. We started our hike where the Appalachian Trail crosses Petites Gap, near the Blue Ridge Parkway in Virginia. We could see the neighboring ridgeline through the naked trees. The forest floor was blanketed with different shades of leaves worn down since the fall. A few brave bloodroot shoots peeked out from the damp soil.

I followed Horton's long gait and plodding feet. He carried an axe over his shoulder. I smiled, thinking that this was probably how my mother first envisioned me backpacking, heading into the forest with a strange man wielding a large, primitive weapon. I had a pair of three-foot-long loppers in my right hand and figured I could at least put up a decent fight.

We hiked an almost three-mile section that Horton had maintained since 1995. There weren't any "blow downs"—fallen trees across the path—nor was there much brush to clear from the path, so we made work for ourselves. Together we rolled a decaying thirty-foot log a foot farther away from the trail. And we took time to cut down a vine that was almost out of reach of our long arms.

In between the trivial improvements, we laughed and talked. Horton took me off trail to a viewpoint that only he knew about. When we passed other hikers, Horton—in the months leading up to what is surely one of the most contentious presidential elections in U.S. history—yelled out to individuals and groups, asking who they were voting for come November. Which of course meant I spent a lot of time apologizing and hiding behind trees. After we covered his section, we cut through the forest on a route that was only barely discernible in the surrounding ground cover. Horton called it the "No Name" Trail. It was hidden from the untrained eye, and we followed it along the headwaters of a crystal clear mountain stream.

As we hiked downhill toward the Blue Ridge Parkway where my car was parked, Horton suddenly tripped, and instinctively released his axe before somersaulting right up to my feet. He stood up as quickly as he'd gone down and wiped the dirt and leaves off his pants and shirt.

"That was close, wasn't it?" he said.

"It's always an adventure," I replied.

Horton is a man of faith, insecurity, and endurance. He is not what I would call graceful. But he has also covered more miles than anyone I know, and I'm not convinced that the two don't go hand in hand. I don't know anyone who's inspired more people to discover the trails or enter an ultra race than this clumsy, flat-footed running machine. He founded an outdoor community in Lynchburg, Virginia, that no one knew was there, and he discovered something extraordinary inside himself despite his self-doubt.

I had always associated David with Dr. Seuss's story about Horton the elephant incubating someone else's egg. But recently, I'd been lying in bed with my daughter reading a different account of Horton, which could be just as appropriate.

In *Horton Hears a Who*, the same caring elephant who'd hatched the egg now hears an invisible voice. And he believes the voice is a sign of life, even though his friends turn on him and think he's deranged. They try to destroy the unseen community that Horton believes in while he does everything in his power to protect it. Eventually, the naysayers hear the voices, too, and realize that Horton was right. There *was* something there.

Endurance is about trusting the invisible voice you believe in, even if nobody else does. Because there's just as good a chance as not that something's really there.

CHAPTER FOUR

The Self-Taught

"What's the point—if I'm not finding personal satisfaction
in what I'm doing?"

—Scott Williamson

David Horton is a legend, but the man who broke his record on the Pacific Crest Trail is a legend among legends. Even among fastest-known-time athletes and elite long-distance backpackers, Scott Williamson is in a league of his own. At age forty-four, Scott has backpacked more than fifty-five thousand miles of long-distance trails. He was the first to complete a yo-yo on the Pacific Crest Trail (meaning he hiked all the way from Mexico to Canada and when he reached the Canadian border, he turned around and hoofed it back to Mexico). He's hiked the trail twice in the same calendar year—and he's done *that twice*, first in 2004 and again in 2006.

Scott has also set and reset the fastest known time on the Pacific Crest Trail three times. He first set the FKT in 2008 when he completed the trail in seventy-one days with his friend Joe Kisner. The following summer he teamed up with another buddy named Adam Bradley, and together they lowered the previous record by several days. Two years later Scott went back by himself and brought the mark down again. This time he hiked southbound from Canada to Mexico in sixty-four days—an average of 41.6 miles per day—during one of the biggest snow years on record.

It's fair to say that while it's possible for you to set a record with Scott, it is unlikely that he'll let you keep it. I can only imagine the blend of pride and frustration that Joe and Adam must have felt when their good friend and hiking partner subsequently broke the mark they had worked to set together. I bet they were thinking, if not audibly saying, "C'mon, man! Don't you remember how deep we had to dig for that? The lightning storms, encounters with mountain lions, and hours of night hiking we faced together? Can't you just hold off a few years and let someone else break it first?"

But to know Scott is to know that year after year he'll return to the Pacific Crest Trail to test his limits.

He's covered more than 80 percent of his miles on the West Coast trail; he's spent more time there than he has inside his house. But Scott has also trekked countless shorter routes and the triumvirate of long-distance hiking: the Pacific Crest Trail, the Appalachian Trail, and the thirty-one-hundred-mile Continental Divide Trail through the Rockies, which together are known as the Triple Crown. Scott's resume includes solo adventures and treks with partners. He has mastered traversing the desert in summer and snow covered mountains in the winter. One can easily make the argument that he is the most talented and experienced long-distance backpacker in the world. He has so much experience, so many stories to share.

The only problem, at least for me, is that Scott Williamson shares his stories with very few people.

Scott Williamson has responded to a small number of media requests since 2004. He has felt exploited and misrepresented by past articles, and that has left a bad taste in his mouth, which leads him to decline most inquiries today. Because he doesn't make his living from hiking or endorsements, he has nothing to gain from publicity. Rarely does a person forsake society for the wilderness for months or even years at a time because he's seeking out the limelight.

Yet Scott's story is foundational in the development of FKTs. Much of the ethos surrounding trail records is derived from the standard that he set. His approach to hiking captures the spirit of amateurism and devotion to purism that defines a sport Scott unknowingly—and perhaps unwillingly—helped to fashion. Whether he likes it or not, Scott Williamson embodies the essence of trail records.

I wanted the opportunity to get to know him. I was hoping to hear even just a few of his countless trail stories. And as someone who was interested in understanding endurance and documenting the history and the spirit of fastest known times, I knew that a conversation with Scott was pivotal if not imperative. But before I could hope to talk with him, before I could try to win his trust, first I had to find a way to get in touch with him.

It's easier to find Scott Williamson on the trail than to reach him by email or phone. Getting hold of him is not unlike contacting a Buddhist monk in some remote monastery in Outer Mongolia.

I started my ill-fated efforts by reaching out to another Pacific Crest Trail record holder. That individual did not have his well-guarded contact information, but she did have an email address for his wife, Michelle, and said she would pass along the project overview to her on my behalf.

Then she added, "I hope Scott will participate. I know he's been burned by media and isn't too keen on it anymore, but fingers crossed . . ."

Several days later I received an email from Michelle, who said, "Sounds like a great opportunity. I'll forward it to Scott and if he's interested he'll send you an email." (I would later learn that this is *verbatim* the email that she sends to everyone who wants a piece of Scott's time.)

At first, I felt optimistic.

A week passed and I held out hope.

Then two weeks went by and I began to assume that I wouldn't hear from Scott.

But, on day fifteen, I received a reply.

I opened the email with trepidation. Somewhere amid the niceties my eyes fell on the humble reply, "I suppose I have a few things to say . . . but who knows if any of it is of any real value. Let me know if you would wish to get together at some point."

A smile spread across my face. I looked up from my computer and stared out the window toward the distant mountains. I was headed west . . . to see Scott Williamson. He'd decided to trust me with his story.

Then it sank in and my smile steadied into a flat horizon. I was going to spend time with Scott Williamson. He was going to trust me with his story. And, now, I had the responsibility of not letting him down.

A few weeks later I boarded a plane for Reno, Nevada. When it landed I strapped on my backpack, walked past the blinking slot machines in the airport terminal, and strode into the cool, crisp air at the foot of the Sierra Nevada Mountains. Within minutes Scott and Michelle pulled up and stepped out of their car to greet me with a hug.

The process of contacting Scott was filled with anxiety, but in his presence I immediately felt welcomed and at ease. His strong jaw line created an imposing presence, tempered only slightly by his wise eyes and the earnestness of his voice. He had the build of a man who cuts down trees with a thirty-five-pound chainsaw, not some emaciated hiker who puts in forty-mile days and survives on refried beans and corn chips.

Michelle sported strawberry-blond pigtails and a grin framed by girl-next-door freckles. A healer who specialized in traditional Chinese medicine, acupuncture, and Qigong, her radiant spirit intimated her holistic practice. She was a physical and—as I would soon witness—emotional counterbalance to her husband.

On our drive out of the valley, I asked Scott why after years of silence he agreed to share his stories with me.

"I mean, you did read the part of the email that said I wanted to write about you, right?!" I had just flown across the country for this meeting, and I still felt compelled to lightheartedly give the man one last out.

Scott smirked. "I agreed because you're a hiker," he said succinctly. Then he fell silent.

I looked out the car window at the snow-covered mountains. I struggle with my confidence as an author. I assume that my assignments have more to do with my miles than my prose. But in that moment, I realized that if it were the other way around, if I were more of a writer than a hiker, I wouldn't be in the car with Scott. We had not shared any miles, but we shared trails and experiences. We were coming from the same place. Being a hiker got me to places that an average writer couldn't go.

A few seconds passed and Scott added, "Plus, you were willing to travel out here and spend time with us. Most people just want to do a quick phone call, then they create click bait."

Michelle took one hand off the steering wheel and rested it on Scott's forearm. "He gets so many inquiries," she said. "And everyone wants something without giving anything in return. I try to filter all of Scott's emails so he doesn't have to deal with it. I pass many messages on to him and he never writes back. But I was hoping he would write you. What he's done is important. It needs to be recorded by someone who understands."

Shifting in his seat, Scott interjected, "I really don't know how much I have to contribute. Everything I know, everything I've learned on the trail, I've picked up from other people."

Scott was being unnecessarily humble, but he also expressed a sentiment that I had heard and experienced time and again. Hikers have two primary teachers: nature and other hikers. When I set out on my first thru hike, I spent countless hours and miles talking with men and women, young and old. From those interactions I learned to identify plants and birds and I discovered new gear and backpacking hacks, but I also internalized people's deepest regrets and greatest sources of pride.

When a retiree looks back at his life and tells you what he would do differently, you listen. When a young child tells you what she loves most about her mother, you take note. My next teacher is always just around the bend.

After a breathtaking thirty-minute drive, we pulled up to Scott and Michelle's home in Truckee, California. Truckee is a resort town located a few miles north of Lake Tahoe where the median home price is more than half a million dollars. The affluent vacation destination of Bay Area techies is not where Scott, a blue-collar arborist who spends as many months on the trail as on the job, thought he might settle. But he lives here to commune with his mountains and with Michelle, who started a practice here in 2004.

Together, they welcomed me into their rental house and introduced me to their two long-haired cats. Most serial hikers don't have pets and I was surprised to learn that Scott Williamson was a cat guy.

Michelle explained that she knew Scott was special when her last cat took to him immediately.

"My kitty's name was Sunshine," she said. "But Scott named him Bink soon after meeting him because he was cuddly like a Binky."

It took a minute for that to sink in. Scott, the reclusive tree feller and mountain dweller, named the pet Bink because he was cuddly like a Binky.

I couldn't help but wonder if Bink was truly drawn to Scott, or if the feline was captivated by the forest scent that permeates his clothing. (My silent suspicions were later strengthened when I learned that Scott owned only one set of clothes at the time he and Michelle started dating.) Regardless, the connection and affection was mutual. Scott was so fond of the cat that after years of going by his real name on the PCT, he took Bink as his trail name. And when their beloved pet passed, Scott buried him in an undisclosed location beside the Pacific Crest Trail.

"He actually did his speed record in 2011 for Bink," said Michelle. "He knew that he was getting old and going to pass soon. Every time I talked with him on the phone he said, "I'm doing it for Bink!"

My higher power was One God, Father Almighty, Maker of Heaven and Earth. Scott's was a cat.

I sat down at the dining room table while Michelle put away groceries and Scott tended the wood stove that heated their cabin. The setting was cozy and peaceful. There were books lining the walls, the fire started to crackle nearby, and on the stove a kettle steamed for our evening tea. But I couldn't fully relax.

I'd asked Scott if we could take a hike during my visit, but keeping up with him now seemed unlikely. Scott was planning to go after the PCT record again that summer and was already in incredible physical condition. Meanwhile, my training consisted of putting in sixty-hour weeks at my home office and taking care of my four-year-old daughter. In other words, I was lucky to fit in a three-mile run every few days. How was I going to keep up with Scott in the high-elevation snow fields of the Sierra Nevada Mountains?

The next morning, I walked out of my bedroom, donning my most technical gear and my best game face. When I entered the kitchen, I saw Scott kneading bread and Michelle chopping vegetables and bacon in the kitchen. I guess the plan was that he would feed me, then crush me.

We enjoyed a leisurely brunch, but with only a few bites of quiche remaining on my plate, I broke down and confessed my fears about hiking with Scott.

Scott looked at Michelle and let out a soft laugh. "Don't worry," he said, "I never train on the weekends when I'm working. Standing on a climbing gaff to cut down trees is much harder than hiking eighteen-hour days. I get all the exercise I need and then some at work. On the weekends, I just try to recover."

I was relieved and also intrigued. It was striking to hear someone who had set so many trail records complain about the physical toll of his work. It was also strange that someone who loved the outdoors made his living cutting down trees.

"Do you like your job?" I asked.

"I loathe it," he said. "I don't mind cutting down dead or hazardous trees. But in Truckee most of the trees we clear are for view enhancement and lot development. We just cleared out a plot of land to create building sites for ten-thousand-square-foot vacation homes." He looked up at me and repeated, "Ten-thousand-square-foot *second* homes, called *eco-cabins*."

Scott pulled out a photo album and pointed to pictures where he is standing in a tree, wearing a hard hat, and holding on to a chainsaw that is nearly as tall as he is. He went on to tell me that if it was not for work—and his wood stove—he would never touch a chainsaw. He conceded, however, that the job did provide decent money, enough money to go hiking each summer. He also said that his boss was an okay fellow, who didn't mind if he left for several months each year. That's a pretty big perk for a long-distance hiker.

But even as Scott rehashed the benefits of his trade, he started to gently rotate his left wrist and stretch out his fingers with a slight grimace on his face.

"I have carpal tunnel in both arms, and my body is so exhausted after several days of work that I have to spend the entire weekend lying on my back to recover. I've been doing this since my twenties," he said. "But I can't do it much longer. It's killing me."

"What else would you do?"

"I don't know," he said. "But hiking from 4:00 a.m. to midnight seems a lot more natural to me than waking up and going to a job that I wouldn't have if it didn't involve a paycheck."

And with that, he stood up, cleared our empty plates from the table, and began washing them in the sink.

After brunch—and after Scott spread bird seed across the

banister of his porch to feed the Steller's jays, crows, and cardinals that greeted them each morning—the three of us decided that we would head to Sierra City for a seven-mile hike on the PCT, below the snowline and up to the base of the rugged Sierra Buttes.

On our drive to the trailhead, Michelle told me that when Scott was a little boy he would climb into tall trees and refuse to come down.

"It used to infuriate his dad," she said. "He couldn't do anything to get him out of a tree. Scott would climb up in the afternoon and not come down till after dark. Eventually his dad decided to just leave him up there and go home."

As we drove through the small town of Sierra City, population 221, memories of my Pacific Crest Trail hike came flooding back to me. I could see myself as a twenty-three-year-old resupplying at the general store and eating dinner on the patio behind the small brick restaurant. I remembered sitting at the far end of a wrought-iron table and ordering a salad. I had hiked close to forty miles that day, and I ordered a salad. It wasn't filling, but I was so sick of energy bars and jerky that I just wanted something fresh. I'd hiked through Sierra City more than ten years ago, but my experiences on the trail were still vivid.

The same was true for Scott. When we started our hike toward the Sierra Buttes, he had a new story at every switchback. He pointed to a forest service road that crossed the blacktop several miles from town and explained that when he'd set the record in 2011, a man driving a jeep had stopped him there and hollered out the window, "Hey, we ran out of beer. You got any extra?"

Scott looked over both shoulders to make sure the man wasn't talking to someone else. Seeing nothing behind him but the thin straps of his ultralight backpack, be turned back to the man and replied, "No."

The man seemed dejected but stayed persistent, "Are you sure? You don't have a thirty rack, do you?"

"I just looked at the man, befuddled," Scott said. "I put my palms out to show him I was empty-handed, shrugged my shoulders, and shook my head. He just sped off and I kept hiking."

Scott's reenactment combined with the thought of his carrying thirty cans of beer in a minimalist pack—and on a record hike, no less—had me stumbling down the trail with laughter.

As it turns out, Scott's not always a masochist. When he and Michelle go backpacking with their friends, they don't hike very far. Plus, Scott will often fill up a large pack with incentives like cold drinks and a cast-iron skillet for cooking steak and asparagus. Unsurprisingly, his close friends have come to really enjoy their outings together.

As we walked, he described the changes to Sierra City over the past ten years and explained the history of the region, which included heavy deforestation and mining. When I pointed out what I thought was an old roadbed, Scott corrected me and said it was a defunct culvert that once directed snowmelt and rainfall downhill to a nearby logging operation. He also described in detail the significance of the region to the California Gold Rush, sheepishly admitting that he had spent far too many hours sifting through old creek beds with his hands, looking for gold flakes.

"I wouldn't do it," he said, "except occasionally, I find one. I have about a hundred hours invested in a tenth of an ounce of gold."

When the trail reached a viewpoint, Scott would name and describe each distant peak before offering me his oversize binoculars for a close-up view. Scott could identify every variety of tree in the forest and could approximate their age. He also knew exactly which switchbacks had a side trail that led to a cold stream. Together, we filled our bottles and drank the unfiltered spring water. It was good to taste the PCT again.

As we neared our car parked at the trailhead, I turned to Scott and asked a question that had been answered throughout the hike, but I still wanted to see if he could put it into words.

"Why do I hike?" Scott repeated to himself. "My experience with hiking is that it's absolutely an experience not found anywhere else in my life. Being in nature, feeling completely at peace, feeling at ease . . . when I'm out there, I feel right."

Scott Williamson is one of the most intelligent and introspective individuals I've ever come across, despite the fact that he never graduated from high school.

He admits that "high school for me was a complete disaster. I missed a lot of school and got kicked out several times."

Then he continued, "It just wasn't stimulating. It was boring. A lot of times I skipped and went to Richmond Public Library to read. I actually thought the books at the library were a hell of a lot more interesting than the textbooks they were using at the public high school."

Richmond, California, is east of San Francisco Bay. In the early 1940s it was home to four shipyards built to meet the high demand for ocean freighters and carriers during World War II. Laborers were brought in from all over the United States, the majority of whom were African Americans who arrived from the Midwest and Southeast by train.

Once the war ended, Richmond had a surplus of tradesmen and a dearth of jobs. As industry declined, drug use and gang violence increased.

"I grew up in an extremely violent environment," Scott said. "Crime rates were among the highest in the country. There was easy access to weapons and drugs. And I became well acquainted with racial divides and discrimination."

As a boy, Scott remembers vividly the time two young men broke into his house while his family was home. His dad, a career machinist and an imposing physical presence, managed to apprehend the burglars, pinning them both down on the floor. Then, with his knees in their chests, he told them in no uncertain terms *never* to come back. Scott's father is now in his seventies. But the way Scott tells it, you still wouldn't want to cross Dave Williamson.

"When it comes to confrontation, my father is old school," Scott said.

Michelle put it even more succinctly: "He'll kick your ass."

When Scott was a child, Dave spent long hours at work, trying to support his family and provide a good life for his kids. Scott loved his dad; he admired his toughness and his tireless commitment to job and family. But Dave's demanding work load meant that most of the time Scott was in the care of his mother—a mother who struggled with mental illness. And she was incapable of properly caring for herself, let alone her children.

When Scott speaks of his mom, he reveals both empathy and injury. It is clear that even though she has passed, Scott still wants to protect her, or perhaps guard his father, who loved her dearly. But he readily and firmly admits, "She abused me emotionally."

Maybe that's why as a preadolescent, Scott would climb trees and refuse to come down. Or why he would ride his bike to Wildcat Canyon and spend the day exploring the creek beds and trails, returning home only after dark, covered in mud and poison oak. Maybe Scott spent his high school years at the Richmond library because it felt safer and more stable than school—or home.

I wonder—perhaps Scott does, too—how much of his tendency for escapism, whether into nature or into books, was a result of his innate disposition and how much was the abusive environment he found himself in. It is, of course, a question that is difficult, if not impossible, to answer. Still, it's undeniable that as a child, Scott was surrounded by bad influences at almost every turn. Fortunately, one of those bad influences introduced Scott to backpacking.

When one of Scott's buddies was convicted of burglary at age ten, as part of his sentencing, juvenile court forced him to join the Boy Scouts. Scott, being a good friend, decided to tag along to the local meetings. His counterpart quit as soon as he'd served his time, but

Scott remained active in Scouts for the next eight years. By the time he was eighteen, Scott had not only earned the coveted Eagle Scout award; he had also discovered a community that provided structure, strong role models, and access to the outdoors.

In 1990, when Scott was sixteen, his troop set out on a fifty-mile backpacking trip through the Sierra Mountains. The group was forced to turn back the first day when one of the leaders suffered a mild heart attack.

Having to help someone you know well out of the woods while he is in cardiac arrest would be enough to keep most people at home indefinitely. Scott and a friend decided to go back and attempt the section on their own.

The route that they traveled followed the Pacific Crest Trail from Mosquito Pass to Echo Lake Resort. During that stretch they met backpackers who were out to complete a seven-hundred-mile portion of the PCT, a trail that Scott would soon learn was more than twenty-five hundred miles long.

The length of the trail captivated Scott. He began searching for books in the library about long-distance hiking and became inspired by adventure memoirs like *The High Adventure of Eric Ryback* and *Journey on the Crest* by Cindy Ross. Scott knew that you could run away to the woods; he had been doing that since he was a young boy. What he didn't realize was that you could live there for months at a time.

The following summer Scott went back to the PCT, this time to hike 241 miles from Lake Tahoe to Yosemite National Park.

The next year, he went back again. He took a bus from Richmond to Southern California and then caught a ride to a small town called Campo, a map dot of border guards, drug smugglers, hardworking immigrants, and aspiring long-distance hikers. Scott touched the PCT monument and started hiking north with an eighty-pound pack on his back. After a few days on the trail, he developed an inflamed Achilles tendon and was forced to stop. He took a Greyhound bus to Los Angeles, then boarded a second back to Richmond.

As he left the downtown Los Angeles bus terminal, he heard a commotion outside. Looking through the enormous glass window he saw angry mobs filling the streets, pushing, yelling, shoving, and throwing anything and everything into the air. He could hear sirens in the distance and he watched as the bus slowly navigated through the crowds, trying to escape the first throes of what would become the L.A. riots, the violent civil protest that led to fifty-five deaths and more than a billion dollars in damage.

When he arrived home, he went straight to his doctor, who inspected his Achilles and promptly informed him that there was no way in hell he could continue hiking that summer. But Scott was already second-guessing his decision to come off the trail. His reintroduction into society had been met with riots, and the pain of being in Richmond felt worse than a strained Achilles. "I rested for about a week," he said. "After that, I remember thinking to myself, *screw it.*"

So he lightened his pack, bought another bus ticket, and returned to the Southern California desert to resume hiking. In spite of his trip to and from Richmond and the nagging injury, Scott managed to hike the length of California that summer. But he still wasn't sated.

He worked through the winter, then went back to the trail—not to Ashland, Oregon, where he'd left off the previous year, but back to Campo. He started walking from there and didn't stop until he made it to Canada. And at the age of nineteen, Scott walked the entire 2,663-mile PCT. These days it's estimated that more than five hundred people complete the trail each year, and the number is growing. But in 1993 only thirty-two people did it.

"I wasn't the same person after that," said Scott. "I came home and started throwing away everything I owned. My parents thought I was crazy. The trail taught me what I needed and what I *didn't* need. I learned a lot—how to take care of my feet, find shelter, regulate food, and stretch finances. I learned to live; I learned how to take care of myself."

When he was twenty, Scott completed the Continental Divide

Trail, a remote and often undefined thirty-one-hundred-mile route. The CDT follows the spine of the Rocky Mountains and, like the PCT, travels between Mexico and Canada. Scott was one of only two thru hikers to complete the trail that year.

The following spring, he made his way to the Everglades and hiked the Florida Trail, which travels the length of the Sunshine State through cypress swamps filled with alligators and water moccasins. When he reached Georgia, he followed the blue highways beside countless pickup trucks to arrive at the southern terminus of the Appalachian Trail. After completing the entire AT and finishing at Katahdin, he decided to continue hiking toward Canada. Scott was stopped forty-three miles south of the border by a private logging operation that wouldn't let him continue across company land. Looking back, there's bitter irony in the fact that professional tree cutters were the ones who stopped Scott Williamson from reaching the border.

At the age of twenty-two, he had already covered twelve thousand miles of long-distance trails. It wasn't a four-year degree, but Scott Williamson was getting an education.

"How did you pay for your hikes?" I asked.

"Most of the early trips were financed by plumbing and construction work, along with a part-time job at a liquor store," he said.

"Wait," I interjected, "weren't you too young to work at a liquor store between those hikes?"

Scott laughed. "I worked at a liquor store before I was old enough to legally sell or drink the stuff."

In 1996, he was working as much as he could, saving up for yet another PCT adventure. Several months earlier, he had attended a hiker gathering put on by ALDHA West—a spin-off of the Appalachian Long Distance Hikers Association that Warren Doyle helped found back east. The weekend workshop is like a much smaller, dirtier version of Comicon. It's a time for an impassioned subculture to geek out together. During a casual conversation at the conference, the seed had been planted in Scott's mind that the trail could feasibly be hiked *twice* in the same calendar year. He was determined to make it happen. Scott wanted to be the first person to "yo-yo" the PCT.

So when his boss at the liquor store called on Sunday, January 20, and asked him to work the four-hour afternoon shift, Scott willingly agreed even though he hadn't been on the schedule that day.

The store was a fairly quiet one. Scott spent most of his hours reading *The New Yorker*. Around 4:30 p.m., his friend James came in to keep him company until he got off work at five.

It was almost quitting time when Scott looked up from his magazine and noticed a man dismounting his bike just outside the plate-glass window. Probably buying a postwork bottle for him and his buddies, Scott thought. The man walked into the store and straight to the counter where Scott was standing.

He was wearing a hoodie and was staring down at the floor, so Scott couldn't see his face clearly.

"What time is it?" The man asked without looking up.

Scott glanced at the clock on the register. "Four-fifty," he replied.

The man was fidgeting with something in the large front pocket of his sweatshirt. Scott figured he was digging for his wallet. Then, in a split second, the man yanked his arm out and pointed a gun at him.

"I saw his face briefly," Scott said, "and heard him mumble something. I think he said, 'I'll shoot you, motherfucker.' Then the gun went off . . . I felt a wave of force hitting me, light and heat—like I was being hit by a train that was on fire. It knocked me sideways and onto my knees. I knew I'd been shot. I jumped up and ran to the back of the store."

The gunman followed.

The storage room had a back door with access to the street. But it was locked. The only key for it was kept up front by the cash register, and for security reasons, the door frame had recently been reinforced with steel casing. Scott tackled the door, using his shoulder as a battering ram. He ripped the door from its hinges, knocking it out of the exterior wall—then he kept running.

But the gunman kept shooting. Bam . . . bam bam . . . bam bam bam. In all, seven rounds were fired at Scott, close enough to singe his hair and burn his shirt. He had felt the heat and the force of the bullets so intensely that he wasn't sure if they'd hit him or barely missed. He sprinted four blocks, then turned the corner to find a mother and her son bringing groceries into their house. Through his mangled jaw, Scott asked for help. The family herded him into their home and locked the door.

"They kept asking me 'Is he behind you?! Is he behind you?!' Then the woman and her son loaded a magazine into an automatic pistol. It was surreal. The son called to another brother in Spanish and he came into the room with a *shotgun*. I remember lying against the wall. There was this immense pool of blood forming beneath me on the floor. I just kept apologizing. I told them I would take care of it."

But the gunman wasn't following Scott. He'd gone back to the store, where Scott's buddy James, who had been in a different part of the store and out of sight during the shooting, was still trying to figure out what had happened.

When the gunman reentered the liquor store, he immediately cornered James. With his hands up, James offered him money. But the man wasn't there for money.

He pushed his would-be victim against the wall. James could see the man's teeth had been filed down. He said they looked like the teeth of a vampire. The man pointed his gun at James's head and pulled the trigger.

But the gun didn't discharge. It was jammed.

James lunged at him and tried to wrestle the gun away, but the man in the hoodie pointed the gun at the back of James's head and fired again. This time the gun went off. James was shot point-blank in the back of the head, but miraculously, he wasn't mortally wounded. On the contrary, he kept fighting and eventually managed to pull the gun away, turning it on his assailant. Then he pressed the trigger. Click. He tried again . . . and again. Click. Click. The gun was empty.

Without any bullets, he grabbed the man in the hoodie and pressed the gun to his forehead. The tables were turned and the man now looked at James in terror. To keep the assailant on edge, James continued to pull the trigger as he backed him out of the store. When they reached the entrance, the man with the teeth like fangs ran for his bike and rode away.

Leaving a trail of blood behind him, James stumbled to a pay phone and called 911.

The bullet that had hit Scott went through his jaw and lodged itself in his uppermost vertebra. Doctors said if the gunshot had been a quarter of an inch higher or lower, he would be a paraplegic. The bullet was never removed.

Scott was released from the hospital after three and a half days. But the impact of the bullet left him bruised from the waist up. What's more, he worried that he might never look normal again.

"My face was blown up and my jaw was held together with wire. I felt like the elephant man," he said.

The gunshot that struck James blew a piece of his skull into his brain cavity. But it never got past the dislodged bone. His brain and his life had been spared. He was released from the hospital ten days later.

Scott has no idea what happened to the man who shot them. "Because no one died, the police didn't spend too much time on it," he said. "There was a Hispanic man who was killed in a gang incident a week or so later. The detectives showed us his picture and told us that this was the man who had shot us. But James and I both said it wasn't the guy."

There is a commonly held notion that people who hike two thousand plus miles are doing so to escape something or to run away. Still others think folks who take a long walk are in need of emotional healing or trying to fill a spiritual void. Those theories are often true. But there are also many people who, like Scott, simply enjoy walking in nature.

On March 3, 1996, forty-two days after being shot, Scott began his yo-yo attempt on the PCT. Most would think it unwise to head into the backcountry for a long-distance hike, let alone a PCT yo-yo attempt, after suffering a bullet wound to the head. But for Scott, the start date couldn't come soon enough. He didn't take a walk because he was shot, but it wasn't going to derail his plans either.

He left the Pacific Crest Trail's southern monument with his best friend, Kenny. Together they planned to return to the same monument, on foot, later that fall.

Scott and Kenny met on the PCT in 1993. Their hiking styles and personalities were compatible and they became fast friends and hiking partners. They finished the trail together, hiking roughly eighteen hundred miles side by side.

Like Scott, Kenny had been training and saving his money for their yo-yo. They had both spent hours constructing lightweight camping gear and strategizing food drops. They knew that in theory the hike was possible and they believed they had the physical capacity and mental fortitude to make it happen. But what they didn't have was the ability to glean knowledge from someone who had gone before. There was no guidebook for hiking the trail twice in a calendar year. They were on a marked trail, but they were in completely uncharted territory. They were pioneers. Their primary teacher would be trial and error.

"We made a lot of mistakes," Scott said. "We started too early. There was too much snow. Forty-three miles north of the border we ran into four feet of it. We expended too much energy dealing with that."

Hiking high mileage days on snowshoes and carrying winter gear would be difficult for anyone. But Scott had an especially rough go of it because he was still struggling to chew.

"I could hardly take in food," he said. "I had limited range of motion in my jaw and it hurt to eat."

Despite the poor conditions, the two arrived at Kennedy Meadows, seven hundred miles north of the border, on April 1. When they got to the outpost that marks the start of the high Sierras, neither man had eaten anything for two days. They had been delayed by storms on the last section, and they came dragging into the resupply point completely depleted.

Scott's father, Dave, was waiting for them with a truck bed full of food. Scott remembers his dad watching in disbelief as Kenny put down three pounds of potato salad in a matter of minutes.

After eating and resting for two solid days, they ventured into the Sierra Nevadas. They didn't take a tent with them because they knew that every night they would be building a snow cave for shelter. It took them a full ten days to get out from under the shadows of Mount Whitney—the tallest mountain in the continental United States—and arrive at the PCT's high point.

The 13,153-foot Forester Pass is a difficult traverse in the *summer* months, let alone in April, when a thick shroud of white covers any discernible route markings to the ridgeline. After an arduous climb to the pass, in which Kenny took the lead chopping steps into the forty-five-degree slope of rime ice, the two friends reached the saddle and started their descent.

Their steps were focused as they tried to safely and efficiently reach the tree line before nightfall. Scott's eyes were fixed on the rhythmic motion of his crampons when suddenly his feet slid out from under him. Everything in his field of vision was moving; the mountain itself seemed to be sliding downhill.

The top crust of the snow had broken away, and Scott was sailing down the mountain on a three-inch-thick avalanche slab. Somehow he managed to stay upright and was deposited a quarter mile from where he last stood. Loose snow continued to rain down on him, covering his legs up to his waist. Within seconds, it felt as if he were stuck in hardened cement. If the snow had continued to fall, he would have been buried alive.

Kenny was still hundreds of yards uphill. Scott called to him for help, and together they used their ice axes to free him from the paralyzing pressure of compacted snow and ice.

The next day, they hiked over Kearsarge Pass and into the town of Independence, where they took two weeks off to look for work and wait for the snow to melt.

More than six months after they'd struck out from the southern terminus, Scott and Kenny reached the Canadian border on August 10. They spent two hours at the PCT's northern monument, then they turned around and started south. With the snow gone, they were now averaging forty-mile days. After traversing Oregon, again, and reaching the Marble Mountain Wilderness Area in Northern California, again, Kenny mentioned offhandedly that his foot was bothering him. By the time they reached the small town of Castella for their resupply, he could hardly walk.

He went straight to the doctor and discovered that he'd broken his third and fourth metatarsals. He had been walking on a broken foot for nearly a week. "I don't know how he did it," Scott said. "I can't imagine the pain it put him in."

Kenny insisted that Scott go on without him, so he did. After several hundred miles, Kenny rejoined Scott on the trail at Tuolumne Meadows in Yosemite National Park. They made it another 28.6 miles together, then it started to snow—and snow, and snow, and snow...

For eleven days snow fell virtually uninterrupted, accumulating higher and higher on the ground. Scott and Kenny were forced to hole up at Red's Meadow Campground. It was the end of the season and there were no tourists, so they had the run of the place. They spent some of their time sharing meals, snacks, and more snacks with the caretaker, who'd no doubt expected to be all by his lonesome. The rest of their days they relaxed in the meadow's natural hot springs, chatting, resting, and watching the snow fizzle as it hit the steaming mineral water.

After a week and a half, the storm finally broke. They left Red's Meadow hoping to traverse the Sierras on snowshoes. By nightfall, they were back in the hot springs. It had taken them the better part of a day to walk four miles. They accepted the fact that they couldn't safely make it through the mountains. The snow was too deep.

Their yo-yo attempt was over.

Scott could have been deterred by that first failed attempt in 1996. Instead, it made him more determined. It also made him smarter. The following year he started out, solo, at the Mexican border in April. He would have liked for Kenny to have joined him, but by this time his best friend was immersed in whitewater paddling and, as Scott put it, "He didn't have another yo-yo attempt in him." Not many people would.

That year, Scott made it through the southern portion of the trail in better time and with less effort. But he was still held up by late snow in the Pacific Northwest and didn't arrive at the Canadian border until August 18. He decided it was too late in the season to turn around and hike all the way back to Mexico, so he skipped ahead to do some hiking and climbing in the Sierras before returning to work.

While he was, as he put it, "playing" in the Sierras, Scott met some southbound PCT hikers. Because he had nothing better to do and still had food boxes waiting for him along the route, he figured he'd join them for a bit. So he hiked from Vermillion Valley Resort to Mexico, another 900 miles on top of his 2,663-mile thru hike that summer. The flippancy with which he recounts—and nearly forgets—those additional 900 miles provides perspective on just how much time Scott has spent on the Pacific Crest Trail.

He still had unfinished business when it came to completing a yo-yo, but in 1998 he decided to scale back and hike the PCT only once. This time he completed a southbound journey with his then girlfriend.

In 1999, he set out on his third attempt at a PCT yo-yo, but this time he only made it 265 miles. "It just wasn't in my heart," he said. He went home, disassembled his resupply packages, and took off on a road trip to the Pacific Northwest with his girlfriend.

They spent several months climbing over rock and ice on some of the tallest, best-known mountains in the region—Glacier Peak, Mount Adams, Mount Baker, and Mount Rainier. He'd walked hundreds of miles contouring *around* these peaks on the Pacific Crest Trail. Now he was finally climbing up them.

Once they'd had their fill of Washington and Oregon, the duo traveled to the Sierra Nevadas. There Scott climbed all the peaks above fourteen thousand feet, including a summit of Mount Whitney alongside his father. Dave Williamson had always supported his son, but he'd never fully understood Scott's hiking ambitions until that day.

"I think that might have been a turning point with my dad," said Scott. "Maybe he started to think, 'Wow, my son's not a total slacker, because this isn't a Hawaiian vacation out here. There is work involved.'"

And hard work earns Dave Williamson's respect.

By the spring of 2000, Scott was once again single and ready for another yo-yo attempt. This time, he tagged the Canadian border and made it back to California, south of Yosemite National Park, to Vermillion Valley Resort. It was the farthest he had come on a yo-yo attempt. If he could make it 176 more miles, it would put him beyond the highest elevations and dicey weather of the High Sierras, and well on his way to Mexico. Scott left Vermillion Valley Resort, but the early season snowfall forced him to turn back yet again.

Scott had invested more than 12,500 miles in his efforts to claim a PCT yo-yo, without success. Folks in the hiking community were eager to see Scott try again. His hiking credentials earned him respect, but his reputation was centered on a goal he had yet to accomplish. A handful of individuals believed that Scott's success was inevitable; far more thought his attempts were all for naught. Depending on whom you asked, Scott had become a symbol of what was possible—or impossible—on the Pacific Crest Trail. Everyone wanted Scott to prove him or her right. Everyone would have to wait.

After his fourth failed yo-yo attempt, Scott started dating a woman, and together they conceived a child, a girl. The relationship with the woman didn't last long, but Scott very much wanted to be part of his young daughter's life.

"It's hard to talk about," Scott said. "My ex isn't here to defend herself and I don't want to say anything negative about her. There are two sides to every story."

The entire time I was with Scott, I never heard him say anything negative about someone else. Growing up as a Boy Scout, he said that he had a troop leader who never spoke ill of anyone. Scott adhered to this example. He didn't even defame the man who shot him, he simply stated the facts.

But when it came to his daughter and the complicated relationship with his ex, Scott looked up at me with a steeliness I hadn't observed before. And with a sternness in his voice that I wouldn't hear again, he said, "You just need to know this: My daughter is the most important thing in my life."

Sierra Rose was born in October 2001. Because of the strained relationship with her mother and because he was trying to support his father and his own mother, who was wasting away from lung cancer back in Richmond, Scott wasn't able to be there for his daughter's birth. A week after she was born, his mother passed away. Scott didn't hike that year.

Scott did not try for the yo-yo in 2002, but he did spend time mountaineering with his old friend Kenny. And he met Michelle.

When Scott and Michelle met, she was living at a hippie commune. *She* didn't call it that, but she did say quite a few others lived there, including a man who lived on the back porch under a tarp and didn't pay rent. She also told me the tenants weren't allowed to cook meat. And that Lola, the seventy-year-old potter/proprietor, asked Scott—on his first visit to the property, no less—if he would consider being her nude studio assistant. (He said no.)

Michelle lived there while pursuing a degree in acupuncture and traditional Chinese medicine. Meanwhile Scott was biding his time and mending relationships before his next 5,326-mile hike. And in an encounter that can only be described as fate, the man who's never owned a smartphone met the woman of his dreams on an online dating service. (Mind you, this was before dating websites were de rigueur for techies, let alone hippies and hikers.)

Scott was the pick of the week on dreamdates.com, and his profile caught Michelle's attention. On their first date, they talked, took a hike, and didn't leave each other's side for forty-eight hours. Three weeks later, Scott moved into the commune.

Scott was still grieving the loss of his mother and the separation from his daughter. But like shafts of light piercing a dark forest canopy, Michelle brought rays of joy back into Scott's life. Her optimism gave him hope that he would be reunited with Sierra Rose. And that fall Scott's ex agreed to let him attend their daughter's first birthday party.

In early October, he drove to Washington, eager to see and hold his baby girl. But while he was en route, Scott got a call from Kenny's mom asking if he'd seen her son. He hadn't seen or heard from his best friend in weeks, but that wasn't unusual. Like Scott, Kenny had a habit of disappearing into the wilderness. It was one of the things that made the two of them so close.

Scott had been at his daughter's side for three hours when he got another call about Kenny. He was dead, and his death was a suicide.

Scott left the party and headed back to California. His best friend was gone and it would be years before he would get to see his daughter again.

"You know what they don't talk about when someone commits suicide?" Scott asked. "They don't talk about how many lives it fucks up."

"There were five hundred people at Kenny's funeral. And there was a lot of grief. I had lost the best friend and hiking partner I'd ever had, the friend I was most compatible with. It made it difficult for me to form close friendships for a long time. But I felt even worse for his family."

Because Kenny felt like a brother to him, it's no surprise that when *Backpacker* magazine published a 2004 article about Scott, the intro and large swaths of the essay focused on the details of Kenny's suicide. Scott felt betrayed, and he took umbrage at the story. Not only had it reopened a wound, but it also exposed Kenny's suicide—and his still grieving family—to a national audience. The last thing Scott wanted was to bring any more pain to Kenny's parents and siblings. With tens of thousands of miles of backcountry experience, Scott had plenty of material and plenty of captivating story lines. Couldn't the writer have found a different focus?

After that, Scott walked away from whatever limelight he'd been in. He didn't want the attention of the hiking community and he stopped taking media requests altogether.

It isn't necessary to exaggerate Scott's losses and tragedies to amplify his hiking accomplishments. But it wouldn't do justice to his hiking legacy to downplay his struggles or cover up another failure. And that's exactly what happened next.

In his own words, he failed. Again.

In 2003, Scott started another yo-yo attempt. But as soon as he left the Mexican border, the mountains were slammed with late-season snowstorms. He made it to the base of the Sierras, but he knew the mountains he was approaching were impassable, so he quit. He quit the trail and soon after, he also called it quits with Michelle. He'd tried five times to yo-yo the PCT, and every time the failures had seemingly compounded. In the process, he also lost a mother, a daughter, a best friend—and he had just broken up with the one person who had helped him through those losses.

This book is an account of fastest known times, not yo-yo attempts. And it's about trail records, not relationships. But more than miles or feats of athleticism, this is about *endurance*. And sometimes endurance isn't defined by success, but is composed of failures. Scott's personal tragedies and hiking setbacks would be enough to make most folks give up: give up on hope, give up on humanity, and give up on hiking. When it feels as if you are constantly losing and everything good is slipping away, it is difficult to muster the strength to keep trying again and again. But endurance is the ability to continue despite past results and with disregard for future outcomes.

In 2004, Scott left the U.S.–Mexico border on April 20. It was his *sixth* attempt at a yo-yo. On October 27, 191 days after he'd begun, Scott ended his hike at the same monument where he had started. He'd completed the trail twice in the same calendar year. Finally.

On his northbound journey he'd covered most of his miles with a deaf female named Patti Haskins. I asked Scott if he noticed any difference with a female hiking partner. He seemed to think that there wasn't much of a distinction, at least not in terms of his pace or mileage. He said that sometimes they lost time trying to communicate due to Patti's hearing impediment, but their pace and temperaments were compatible.

He hiked by himself on his southbound trip, but managed to mend his relationship with Michelle through handwritten notes and a visit to Truckee.

In the desert, he was forced to wade through knee-high water in arroyos when it rained every day south of the Mojave. But beyond the rain in the desert, there wasn't anything unique about the weather that year. The snow levels in the mountains weren't high then, but neither were they exceptionally low. So what made this go a success?

"I just knew I could do it," Scott said. "I knew it was entirely doable, and it was an uncompleted goal that I had to pursue to the end. There are so many factors out there that are beyond your control . . . the weather . . . injury. But in 2004 it was the right combination of luck and perseverance."

When you have failed over and over again, the decision to keep moving forward is not derived from reason but driven by hope.

Scott Williamson has invested a hundred hours prospecting a tenth of an ounce of gold, and he is the first person to successfully yo-yo the PCT.

He also made the second successful yo-yo of the PCT.

In 2006, Scott attempted the feat once more, and he made it from Mexico to Canada and back again. After that, he was ready for a new challenge.

Scott and Michelle tied the knot. And, as she puts it, "It is challenging to be married to a record setter." As much focus as there is on the individuals who've set fastest known times, their stories can't be fully told without mentioning the support of their partners.

Michelle voiced the same sentiments as Nancy Horton, as she shared how difficult it was to be alone for months at a time. Brew, who sometimes joins me on hikes and other times stays at home, also likes to remind me that it is easier to be the one leaving than the one left behind. But Michelle then added an important afterthought. She said, "Even if being left at home is hard, it is still easier than trying to keep up."

She then flipped through one of Scott's scrapbooks to show me pictures from their honeymoon hike on the PCT in 2007. I looked away when she pointed to a picture of her feet, swollen and soggy from walking, pale with moisture and covered with blisters and bruises. Other snapshots showed Michelle covered in bug bites and clearly fatigued. Meanwhile, Scott stands by her happy as a clam and looking completely unscathed.

"I hiked 650 miles and could not take another step due to my feet being in so much pain," she said. "I had taken eleven Advil that day and it did not touch the pain. Scott brought it to my attention that I was not hiking in the integrity of my beliefs . . . pumping myself full of Western medicine and ignoring the root cause. I agreed, but wanted it so bad. It was a teary night of defeat and pain. I took eleven days off. Scott hiked on. I got back on the trail with him at Seiad Valley. Together we climbed four thousand feet out of the canyon. The next day I woke up gasping for breath . . . it felt like I was sucking air through a straw."

She and Scott immediately got off trail and headed for a nearby town. As soon as they'd stopped hiking, Michelle started to feel better. Scott had taken her breath away in more ways than one. From that point on, they decided it would be better for him to hike the Pacific Crest Trail without her.

Michelle decided to focus on enjoying casual weekend backpacking trips and day hikes with her husband.

She then described an incident that took place several years later, on a day hike near Truckee. Michelle and Scott went for a walk in the national forest and got separated. She'd mistakenly wandered down an old roadbed and wasn't sure where she'd gone wrong. She was wearing a daypack with a few essentials, but she didn't have a map, shelter, or food. She wandered old forest service roads for hours. Eventually the sun started to set, but she could hear vehicles in the distance and she kept hiking. Finally, at dusk, she stumbled out onto a paved highway and spotted the PCT trailhead nearby. She could also see Scott putting the car in reverse and starting to drive away when she came running down the blacktop waving her hands at him.

"What are you doing?" she cried.

"I looked for a while, but couldn't find you, so I figured I'd come back in the morning," Scott said.

"Come back in the morning? You were going to leave me out here? Weren't you worried?!" Michelle shrieked.

"Well, I knew you would be okay because you had a lighter," said Scott.

Scott then gave me an earnest expression to suggest that not only was he justified in his thought process, but I would understand where he was coming from.

Michelle shot me a glance to convey that her husband was an extreme minimalist who placed unreasonable expectations on his wife.

I gave Michelle a nod of compassion.

The year after his honeymoon hike, Scott tried for his first FKT on the Pacific Crest Trail with his friend Joe Kisner, otherwise known as Tatu-Jo.

Covered from head to toe in ink, Tatu-Jo was a long-distance hiker and ultra marathoner who helped Scott concentrate the energy he put toward his yo-yo attempt into a shorter, more sustained effort.

"I learned how to be consistent from him," Scott said. "He taught me how to pace myself. Before that summer, I'd never hiked more than three weeks without taking a zero [day]."

When Scott was trying to accomplish his yo-yo he would take "zero days" (rest days in town when a person hikes zero miles). But on the record hike he had to teach his body to recover in motion.

"So how did it compare?" I asked.

"Setting a record is harder than a yo-yo," he replied, "hands down."

After seventy-one days and with no "zeros," Scott and Tatu-Jo made it to Canada. Together they had set a new unsupported record.

In 2009, Scott went back to try to break his own record, the one he had just set with Tatu-Jo. This time he hiked the trail with a different friend, a man named Adam Bradley.

Adam wanted to break the sixty-six-day supported record that David Horton established in 2005. Scott didn't think it was possible, but he decided to try it anyway.

Horton had masterfully assembled a qualified support team to supply him with companionship, provisions, and an abundance of motivation. Scott and Adam didn't have vehicular support. And whereas most thru hikers hitchhike into town to resupply, they decided that every step of the journey—even their off-trail miles to town and back—would be on foot. Whereas Horton relied on a support van with an ever-changing crew, Scott and Adam relied entirely on each other.

"I think it's much easier to set a record when you're hiking with someone else," said Scott. "It takes away a lot of the mental challenges that come with a record."

What Scott *didn't* mention is that when you try to set an FKT with a partner, you also have to get along with that person, all day, every day, while constantly feeling famished and fatigued. In addition to the added social challenge, partners attempting a record are forced to compromise on pace and mileage to account for whoever is feeling weakest at the time. The fact that Scott has successfully hiked the trail with multiple people, through every kind of trying circumstance imaginable, is a testament to his personality.

As Scott and Adam began closing in on the border, it started to sink in that they were going to break David Horton's record. Or were they?

"We were so tired by the end," he said, "that we didn't know what *day* we were on. It took an entire afternoon for us to figure out if we were going to hit the border on day sixty-five or day sixty-six."

Eventually, the math came together and they realized they were on target to surpass Horton's mark by a full twenty-four hours.

"I felt a little sad about that," he said. "David had become a mythical figure. In my mind, this guy was doing things that I would *never* be able to do. I was bummed that we were going to set that record because I know how hard he had worked to get it. He set the benchmark for these types of endeavors."

Scott and Adam reached the border after sixty-five days. They walked from Mexico to Canada without setting foot inside a car. Their accomplishment surpassed the mark of a fully supported runner—nay, The Runner—who was assisted by a crew and a car. Still, Scott's quick to add, "That experience *vastly* increased my respect for David Horton." I kept trying to ask Scott about his accomplishment, and he kept referencing Horton's. I had known Horton for more than ten years and I owned multiple copies of his memoir and movie. I was hoping Scott could be a little more self-centered with his information.

"You know what's really impressive," said Scott. "Here's a guy who did this when he was fifty-five years old. David Horton will forever hold the master's record on the PCT."

In 2011, Scott hiked southbound by himself and set yet another record, reaching Mexico in sixty-four days. That breaks down to nearly forty-two miles a day with a pack, without company, and never hitching into town.

"What stands out about that hike?" I asked. (Knowing it was a record snow year, I expected him to say something about the difficult conditions, late-season snow fields and high river crossings.)

"Well, I did lose six hours of time helping an injured trail worker.

"I came upon a rider thrown from his horse, a forty-year trail maintainer out of Seiad Valley by the name of Bill Roberts, whom I had met numerous times over the years.

"I walked up on him, his wife, and a section hiker who is a nurse in her regular life, all in the meadow. Bill was on the ground in deep shock. He looked dead to me, an ashen gray color to his skin.

"He had fallen only minutes before I arrived. The other hiker was near them when it happened. She was saying his pelvis was broken.

"I stayed in that meadow for six hours caring for him while his wife ran back to the forest service truck. Then I helped her drive the truck along the PCT tread, weaving between trees and boulders into the meadow where Bill was. We carefully loaded him into the truck.

"There was no cell service. All three of us had different carriers and nobody had any signal. His wife had to drive him off the mountain to call the rescue guys.

"At the time, I thought, well . . . the speed hike is done, I need to help Bill. All I could think is that we have to get Bill to the hospital.

"After they drove off to go meet the helicopter it was 11:00 p.m. I camped nearby. I woke up the next morning at my usual 4:00 a.m. and decided to keep going after it.

"The next day when I arrived in Seiad Valley, I was given word of Bill's condition. After a helicopter ride to the hospital, he was discovered to have a broken pelvis, broken femur, three broken ribs, and a ruptured spleen and bladder.

"Bill knows everyone in that town and is well liked and respected. Word of the scene the day before had preceded me, and no one would accept my money for anything I was trying to purchase. I was treated to a free meal and food and went on my way.

"I was glad I decided to keep going. Even though that six-hour loss threw my timing off for everything the rest of the summer, I still pulled some time off the record."

Scott Williamson, the only person to set a fastest known time on the AT or PCT three separate times—and save a life along the way.

(In a separate feat of endurance, after spending several weeks recovering in the hospital, Bill Roberts went back to trail work at sixty plus years old.)

————————

In 2012 Scott tried for the record again and was stopped by wildfires in Oregon.

In 2013, he made it to California before he discovered blood in his stools and became severely nauseated due to internal bleeding. At the point when he didn't think he could take another step, he was serendipitously able to hitch a ride from one of the trail's most remote access points, some fifty miles from the nearest paved road.

Then, in 2014, the unthinkable happened. Someone broke Scott's record. It wasn't Tatu-Jo, Adam Bradley, or David Horton who lowered the mark. Instead, a woman and a relatively unknown hiker—up until then—named Heather Anderson took four days off the record.

On her journey to Canada, Scott hiked in to meet her and deliver food at Donner Pass.

"I knew she would break the record," said Scott. "There was something about her demeanor, the way she was going about it. I just knew she would get it."

It did not surprise Scott that a woman surpassed his mark. Like Warren, he did not believe that gender was a factor on an FKT. After walking with Patti Haskins on his successful yo-yo hike, he knew that women possessed the stamina to set a record.

"If there was anyone who was going to break the record, I was pretty stoked it was a woman, and it was also a woman who overcame a lot more detractors—for various reasons—than I had. It was redeeming to watch Heather shut those people up. She did it with the style and integrity that I would want someone to do it with."

"Was it hard to let go of the record?" I asked.

"I was a little bummed, but I was elated at the number of days she took off it and that she did it in the same style [without getting into a car]."

"You went after the record after she set it, right? That summer?"

"Yeah, but I wasn't necessarily going after her record. I just wanted to lower my time. I had already planned for a southbound hike that year. But I didn't want to announce it or post anything because I didn't want people thinking I was going after Heather. Plus, I only made it to Oregon that summer.

"Honestly, that's why the past few summers of attempting it, I haven't posted or announced it. I haven't contacted Heather because I have no intention of making it known if I do break her record. So even this summer if I am able to get out there, even if I *were* to best her time, I wouldn't announce it publicly because in my mind it doesn't really matter. It's for me.

"I'm not doing this so people can say, 'Oh wow, you broke the record again.' And in a way, it doesn't matter because as soon as I post it, there's going to be a guy out there next year who breaks it again. What's the point if I'm not finding personal satisfaction in what I'm doing?

"Otherwise, it's not going to motivate me on day forty-five when I'm feeling like shit and waking up to hike when there's still two more hours of darkness. The accolades? That's just not enough. I have to want to do it for myself."

Maybe Scott Williamson will break the PCT record again and maybe he won't. Either way, you and I will never know. But this much is certain: Scott Williamson embodies the true spirit of FKTs.

When I traveled to Truckee to interview Scott, it was the second time that we'd crossed paths. I also met him briefly on my PCT thru hike in 2006. He'd met thousands of people on long-distance trails and we'd encountered each other in the dark of night ten years earlier, but he still remembered our meeting. And so did I.

I'd just gained Egg Butte Ridge in a horrible storm. Heavy gray clouds rushed past me like a raging river. I struggled to stay upright in the strong, cold current. Eventually, I descended out of the clouds with chattering teeth and icicles in the hair framing my face. I looked over my shoulder and noticed the steep drop-offs and precipitous cliffs, which had been hidden by the storm.

I stumbled down the trail in the encroaching darkness to reach Lutz Lake. When I arrived on the shoreline, I was shaken from the storm and shivering from the cold. Overcome with relief and fatigue, I collapsed to the ground and started rummaging through my pack to collect my tent, down sleeping bag, and wool long johns.

I could see that someone else was camping at the far end of the lake. The other hiker was a ways off and I assumed that we would not engage each other. The weather was still unwelcoming, the darkness was spreading, and I didn't have any extra steps in me.

In a few minutes, a lanky guy emerged from the shadows with his headlamp gleaming to greet me. The man introduced himself.

Scott Williamson?!

The beam from my flashlight traveled from his head to the ground and back to his face. His trail reputation preceded him, and I had a hard time believing that I was encountering this mythical hiker in the flesh.

I held him in the spotlight as he stood there and chatted with me. He complimented me on navigating the storm, which I assured him was nothing more than a bad decision mixed with dumb luck. Then he said I was making good time to Canada. He told me that I was one of the few women he'd ever met this close to the Canadian border who was still hiking solo and mentioned that maybe in the future I should consider going for a trail record. I will admit, the fact that Warren and now Scott suggested that I might try for an FKT began to stir my ambition.

Scott then told me that even though Glacier Peak Wilderness was closed due to washouts and flooding, it was passable and he encouraged me to consider taking the route.

The entire time we were together, he talked very little about himself, beyond casually mentioning that his big toe was hurting. And he didn't even hint that he was on pace for his second successful yo-yo. But I knew about it. Everyone on the trail knew about it.

That night I went to sleep, not thinking about the storm that had almost knocked me off the mountaintop, but rather comforted by the kindness and approachability of a man camped on the north side of the lake. The next morning, I walked past Scott's campsite and handed him the remains of my food bag, which consisted of a few random energy bars. I was closing in on a resupply that afternoon. It would be days before Scott hit the next town, and with the onset of winter weather in late August he needed the food more than I did.

A week later, I found myself bear-hugging a fallen tree that spanned a raging river. I was attempting to traverse Glacier Peak Wilderness alone. Salty tears ran into my mouth, along with the cold, sweet rain. As I put my right hand out to take hold of the next broken branch and continue inching my torso across the log, I cursed my decision to enter the closed wilderness.

"What were you thinking?" I yelled aloud. "*You're* not Scott Williamson!"

I vacillate between feeling as if Scott and I are kindred spirits and thinking that he comes from another planet.

I feel connected to Scott, in part because of our miles, but mainly because of our humanity. Most folks would relate to Scott. In fact, it would be hard not to like him. He's spent so much time on the trail with hikers of different stripes that he can connect with almost anyone.

Perhaps the media's real disservice to Scott was in dramatizing him. They magnified his accomplishments and sensationalized his loss. And Scott's decision to decline interviews and withdraw from the public eye allowed the legends to grow.

But if you spend time with Scott, you are left with the impression that he's just an average guy, a blue-collar arborist who struggles to make a living in a mountain town teeming with transplant yuppies. Scott himself says, "For nine months of the year, I don't go around talking about the trail. Most people don't know I'm a hiker." And he likes it that way.

In a way, I am very much like Scott Williamson; we all are. He is an ordinary person. Granted, he is an ordinary person with a backstory that unfolds like a made-for-TV drama. But Scott is not defined by his physical injuries, personal setbacks, and numerous failures. Instead, Scott Williamson has carved out an identity based on his love for the outdoors and a willingness to keep trying—traits that feel both ordinary and attainable.

It's the extent to which Scott has tried, and tried, and tried again, plus the amount of time he has spent in nature, that sets him apart. He has learned lessons that are not readily available in the American public school system or elite institutions of higher learning. He has the wisdom of fifty-five thousand miles of wilderness.

CHAPTER FIVE

The Psychology of Endurance

"Whether you are talking about sports or life in general, the main
thing you are trying to achieve is consistent high performance."

—Dr. Daniel Czech

"The only way we can discover our potential is to test the limits,
to push up and through the boundaries we set for ourselves."

—JPD

In my junior year of college, I signed up for a semester-long
elective called Foundations of Sports Psychology. Our professor, Dr. Daniel Czech, was a proponent of experiential education, so he often incorporated personal challenges and demonstrations
in the lectures.

I'll never forget the day he started class with a wall sit competition. I took my place alongside a dozen or so classmates. We lined up
with our backs to the cool cinder block wall slathered in white paint,
our legs at ninety-degree angles. Dr. Czech started his watch

I closed my eyes and took a long, deep breath. I can't recall what
college coed drama was taking place at the time; I just know that on
that particular morning, I was the right combination of ticked off and
stubborn and I had an edge. Before I ever entered my squat, I was 100
percent sure I was going to outlast everyone else.

I kept my eyelids down and focused on my breathing. I imagined
I was resting in a comfortable leather recliner. Eventually, when my
legs started hurting, I imagined that I didn't have legs at all. One by
one, I gradually said good-bye to the parts of my body that started to
ache. I detached from my feet as they struggled to keep their grip on
the slick linoleum floor, then my calves and quads as the searing pain
radiated up my legs. I disconnected from the pressure in my lower

back, the tingling in my arms, even the pulsing vein in my temple as drops of warm sweat trickled down my nose and fell on my shirt. Within a few minutes, I was entirely in my head.

I could hear other students alternately laughing out loud or crying out in pain. I knew most of them had already pushed off the wall or crumpled to the floor. I could sense that there were only a few of us remaining. I opened my eyes and looked around. There was just one guy left, the star forward on the men's basketball team situated a few feet to my right. I didn't care that he was eight inches taller than me or that his quads were twice the size of mine. I knew he was going down before I did.

I shot him a look—a smirk—that said, "Give up now, buddy. It's no use." (I doubt this is what they are referring to when they talk about making eyes at the opposite sex.) Then I turned my head back, lifted my chin, and closed my eyes again. I released a long, steady exhalation and continued envisioning myself in a comfortable leather recliner. When my body started shaking uncontrollably, I just pretended I was in one of those massaging versions from the Sharper Image catalog.

I signed up to take sports psychology because it was a "soft science" and I assumed it would be an "easy A" that would pad my GPA. But not only was it a challenging course (wall sits were just the beginning), it was also the most influential one I took in undergrad. During the semester-long class, I learned the importance of imagery, goal setting, self-confidence, concentration, and arousal regulation—and no, that's not what you think it is. I also learned I could outlast a basketball jock in a wall sit. And today I use the lessons of sports psychology more than those of any other discipline from my higher-education experience.

When I decided to look into the practices of individuals who set fastest known times, I called my old professor Dr. Czech to get his take. He's now tenured at Georgia Southern University and has spent more than twenty years imparting the importance of sports psychology to his students. The majority of the young men and women who take his class apply the lessons more to their office routine, home life, and hobbies than to bettering themselves or others as athletes. That's probably why he's well known, not just as a sports psychologist but as a professional speaker and business consultant.

Dr. Czech said, "Whether you are talking about sports or life in general, the main thing you are trying to achieve is consistent high performance. You can't operate at 110 percent. It's mathematically impossible. So what we strive to do is enhance our potential on a daily basis, to go from performing at, say, 60 percent, to performing at 80 percent. Then once you accomplish that, the goal becomes *repeating* that higher level of performance."

He went on, "Take Duke's men's basketball as an example. They're always at the top of their conference and the top of the national rankings. You seldom if ever see them at the bottom or even in the middle of the pack. Coach K is *consistently* winning."

As a die-hard Tar Heel fan, that example really irked me. I knew he was right but I would have tweaked his statement. Duke is consistently good enough to give Carolina a run for its money.

Dr. Czech continued, "When you were doing your trail record, you were probably performing at about 90 percent of your potential, not 100. The difference is that you had to do it day after day after day without any breaks and without much rest.

"I'd imagine even now that the record is over you were still trying to reach your potential *off* the trail. And I bet you still want to consistently perform there."

Warren Doyle taught me that an FKT starts with a question, an inner monologue or personal theory about exploration and self-improvement. And since there's no evidence to determine the theory's validity, it nags at and eventually consumes a person until she dares to find out whether the hypothesis is true.

The process is not exclusive to trail records. The need to prove ourselves is human nature. Successes in innovation and exploration are almost always achieved by the people who ask far-fetched questions and then relentlessly pursue the answers. We call it progress. It's one of our unique attributes as a species and it distinguishes us from the rest of the animal kingdom. It can be our glory, our downfall, or both. But whatever it is, it seems to be our destiny. And as much as we may question it or try to repress it, there seems to be an innate drive in society to push farther, to go faster, to build taller and bigger and better.

In the words of the renowned and ill-fated Everest climber George Mallory, "If you cannot understand that there is something in man which responds to the challenge of this mountain and goes out to meet it, that the struggle is the struggle of life itself upward and forever upward, then you won't see why we go."

The psychological origin of trail records is the same as that of almost any far-flung pursuit. As humans, we are intrinsically entranced by possibilities. We wonder if we're capable of more than what we're currently achieving, and the only way we can discover our potential is to test the limits, to push up and *through* the boundaries we set for ourselves.

Endurance athletes are an uncommon breed, difficult to group together and hard to single out in a crowd.

When I spoke with Dr. Czech, he said, "There are definitely distinct personality types that are attracted to certain sports—including extreme sports."

"That's what I thought, too," I replied. "But endurance athletes are all over the map when it comes to personality and background. And I don't think that we're extreme athletes in the traditional sense. I mean, we go extreme distances but we're not like sky divers or base jumpers or free climbers. We're not in it for the adrenaline rush. At least, I'm not!"

Dr. Czech laughed, "You might have different interests and personalities," he said, "but you likely have similar tendencies and motivations. Understanding what motivates people to want to get better or try new things is very important."

Record setters get the "why" question a lot. Even if pushing the boundaries of what is possible is written in the human DNA, it's a wonder that individuals would subject themselves to physical pain, sleep deprivation, and emotional hardship to finish a trail in the shortest possible time frame. It doesn't make sense. It doesn't help anyone. It's not even spectator friendly!

Why not cure a rare disease or excel at a real sport? Why an FKT?

This line of questioning doesn't just come from those outside the trail running and hiking community; a lot of times it comes from insiders, too. And, as record setters, quite often we struggle to come up with sufficient answers.

David Horton said, "It's really hard to explain *why*. In running they say you're only as good as your last long run or race. And I think that's bad. I mean, it's bad in the sense that it's not true. You're not *only* as good as your last race. But I did want to prove something to myself when I went for those records, to myself and to other people."

I don't think that I needed to prove myself on the trail—at least not to other people—but I had an insatiable desire to find out what I could do. Maybe the difference is simple semantics. I didn't have an expectation as much as a curiosity that grew more and more as time passed. I knew if I didn't at least give it a try, I would always look back with regret and wonder "What if?" or "What could have been?" My main reason for starting an FKT wasn't so much a negative question as a positive statement.

I think most FKT athletes struggle to provide a succinct answer to the "why" question because the reasons are too personal to explain. Or maybe too simple to be accepted. If you boil it down, the most basic reason a person goes after an FKT is that he or she wants to, which is a kind of kissing cousin to George Mallory's famous line about why he wanted to climb Everest: "because it's there." The answer isn't complicated; it's just hard to understand.

Perhaps the strongest link between record setters is that we choose to hurt. We sign up for an utter suffer fest—knowing good and well we'll probably fail—because we revel in the waves of endorphins that are released throughout the day, take pride in being the only person on the trail during a driving storm, and delight in the transformation of our pliable bodies into chiseled marble. We also enjoy the sense of progress that comes from taking one more step, walking one more mile, and making it one more day. We all believe that the agony is worthwhile. We have different methods for minimizing and rationalizing the pain, but we all make the decision to suffer.

When you're hiking thousands of miles by yourself for months on end, you have a lot of head space to fill and a lot of pain to ignore. Scott told me that before setting the southbound FKT in 2011, he stopped in a small convenience store in Mazma, Washington, to pick up some supplies. As he selected a couple of snacks and walked up to the cash register to check out, Kenny Rogers's song "The Gambler" was playing over the sound system.

"That song ended up sticking in my head all the way to Mexico," he said. "I can remember so many nights, exhausted, hiking alone in the dark and pushing late into the evening with those lyrics running through my mind. 'You've got to know when to hold 'em, know when to fold 'em. Know when to walk away, and know when to run.' It was torture sort of, but I guess it kept me going. It became my mantra for a while. It's funny now but at the time it drove me nuts!"

One important takeaway from Scott's story is that if you don't choose a mantra, it will choose you.

Case in point: When I was twenty years old, I signed up for an Ironman triathlon. And, yes, Dr. Czech's sports psychology class was partly to blame. At the time, I wasn't a swimmer or cyclist but, like David Horton's students, I had a professor who inspired me to try new things and go farther than I had before.

I bought a bike and started taking swim lessons two years in advance of the race. With so much time, training, and hard-earned babysitting money invested in the event, I wanted nothing more than to do well and finish strong.

Several of my girlfriends traveled with me to Panama City Beach to offer their encouragement and support—and to go to the beach. But I give them credit. On race day, they showed up with bells and whistles on, literally. Every time they saw me they would cheer and yell, ring cowbells and blare rap music, hold up homemade signs and wave pom-poms. As I finished my swim and ran to the bike transition area, one of my friends shouted, "Remember, it's all about the calories." Thinking it was a strange battle cry, I looked over to see her smiling and holding up a poster with the same phrase surrounded by hand-drawn chocolate chip cookies.

I spent the rest of the race daydreaming about all the carbs I was earning and repeating, *It's all about the calories.*

Dr. Czech suggests that the impact of a short phrase on performance is profound. And while there is nothing wrong with repeating Kenny Rogers lyrics or focusing on energy expenditures (and cookies), he encourages his athletes to create mantras based on positive self-talk and affirmations.

"Positive self-talk can help you focus on what you need to do," he says. "If you're constantly focusing on the negatives of past or future events it can keep you from performing to your ability. A mantra can help you overcome that, to trust yourself, control the situation, stay in the present, and work through obstacles. It is a very powerful mechanism."

After exiting the Smoky Mountains with debilitating shin splints, David Horton continued with limited support for several days. He endured a stabbing pain in his lower legs; a heavy load on his back; and when he stopped to pee, his urine was dyed with blood. "This is who I am and this is what I do," he said. "This is who I am. And this is what I do." Then he trudged on, repeating his refrain.

On my AT record attempt, I told myself several times throughout the day, "I belong." When I felt that I couldn't keep up with celebrated runners like Horton or veteran hikers like Warren, I said, "I belong." When I wanted nothing more than to go home and leave the trail behind, I said, "I belong." I have no doubt that those two words helped me traverse two thousand plus miles in record time.

Whether one is going for a trail record, finishing up a big project at work, or trying to make it through the checkout line at the grocery store with a screaming toddler, one can always use a mantra. Identifying positive personal statements is a small, easily accessible measure to help overcome any circumstance. They're not hard to come up with and they don't have to be original phrases.

Warren Doyle has a habit of writing and reciting poetry, so it comes as no surprise that during his FKT he channeled a well-known Robert Frost poem for extra motivation. Late in the day when the beams of light entered the forest at a low angle, when the miles he'd covered left him feeling exhausted and the miles before him left him demoralized, Warren would match the meter to his footfalls and say over and over again, "But I . . . have promises . . . to keep . . . And miles . . . to go . . . before . . . I sleep . . . And miles . . . to go . . . before . . . I sleep."

If you have yet to claim a statement of affirmation, then consider heeding the advice—or adopting the slogan—of the world's largest sports apparel company and "Just Do It."

Even when you are equipped with a mantra worthy of a tea tag, there are still going to be times—times when an opossum gets in your food bag at night and devours all your rations, times when you wake up in a leaking tent to your fifth straight day of rain, times when you unzip the sidewall and discover that one of your hiking shoes has inexplicably gone missing. Yes, there are going to be times when you can't talk yourself through the low points. That's when you pretend you're not there.

Record setters are all about alternative realities.

As David Horton is fond of saying to the thousands of runners who've completed his ultramarathons in Virginia, "It can't always get worse." Despite his mind-boggling terminology, the practical application is simple. Horton likes to imagine himself on the other side of the storm . . . or the mountain . . . or the blackflies. Then he keeps running till he gets there.

On the other hand, his foil and friend Warren Doyle likes to think, "It could always be worse." He envisions the storm getting stronger, the mountain growing taller, or the cloud of blackflies multiplying exponentially until the challenges he's facing start to seem tolerable.

Dr. Czech calls this disassociation. He says it can be a powerful tool, one that athletes most often use when they are dealing with injury. And that makes sense, since record setters are almost always managing injuries—either fending them off or doing their best to handle the hurt.

Whatever you want to call it—disassociation, escapism, denial, or sheer stupidity—endurance athletes use it in spades to cope with the predicaments they find themselves in. We all have the ability to manipulate our thoughts, and sometimes mentally removing ourselves from a situation is the best way to survive it. But be forewarned: The brain likes to play tricks, too.

Scott Williamson shared the following story:

"I was going along one morning at first light and came upon some sort of military vehicle parked about twenty yards off the trail and covered in camo netting. I could see the tires, the thick bulletproof windows, even where the duff had been smashed down when they'd driven in there. I called out to see if anyone was in it, thinking maybe they were doing some sort of training exercise. No one answered. When I left the trail and walked toward it, more of the vehicle's details emerged. I could smell grease and a hint of diesel fuel; I could see through one of the windows. It looked like there was some equipment stacked inside. I couldn't believe it. I mean, I was so confused to see this vehicle parked in such an odd place and so far from a road. I climbed up onto this rock to look into a different window and then just like that, I realized I was looking at a vehicle-sized boulder that was covered in pine needles and tree branches!"

Hallucinations are commonplace during extended athletic pursuits. When you don't get much sleep at night, it's like these insanely vivid dreams have to come out somehow, so they spill out into the middle of the day. It can be almost impossible to tell what's real and what's a figment of your imagination.

I have seen and heard water sources that aren't actually there—particularly when I am dehydrated. I have gone so far as to unscrew the lid of my bottle and bend down to fill it before I realize that there is nothing but dirt and rocks on the ground.

One of my hiking friends thinks he saw a young boy dressed in colonial garb at an Appalachian Trail shelter. He shared a conversation with the child and learned that he was lost and looking for home. The boy starting crying and when the hiker went to comfort him, he disappeared.

A runner I know was so convinced a Sasquatch walked through his or her camp that he or she asked not to be named.

You can't expect a body to cover forty or fifty miles a day without the mind wandering. It can create subconscious renderings, or hallucinations, but with a little focus and imagination you can also sketch a more controlled image. The most common mental picture that we paint on an FKT is the final summit. When you feel that you are only holding on by a thread, that thread is a vision you've dreamed up of what the final mountain will look like.

This form of escapism is different from disassociation. It falls into the category of visualization and is, according to Dr. Czech, the most powerful mechanism we have. "When you use visualization," he says, "you're forming confidence and creating a mental blueprint. There are studies that show a basketball player's free throw percentage will increase if he visualizes making shots. Other research suggests that muscles can actually get stronger *without working out* if an individual will just visualize engaging and exercising those muscles. But just like anything else, this skill has to be practiced."

Record setters are constantly honing this technique. And the closer they draw to the trail's terminus, the more tangible the imagery becomes. You envision walking the final mile with long, fluid strides and you picture the feeling of pride that comes with seeing that last trail sign. You reach out and touch the engraved wood, metal, or stone with your fingers, callused from months of gripping hiking poles or hoisting yourself up jagged boulders. You think about the people who will share the moment with you—your selfless spouse, whom you haven't seen in two months, your crew members, a mother, father, or close friend. You feel their arms wrap around you and you press your weight into them or even fall limp into their arms, able to let your guard down for the first time in weeks.

You wonder about the emotional outbursts that will come with the finish. Will you be crying? Will you howl like a lone wolf, releasing some primal victory call? Or will you simply fall silent because the thunderstorm of emotions is too overwhelming to express? You start to taste food and drink on your lips, something that would be mundane in any other setting but is entirely transcendent in this one. Maybe it's a favorite craft brew a friend brings you from home. Or some celebratory meal—Maine lobster with drawn butter, or cornmeal-crusted mountain trout from a crooked Georgia stream.

When Warren talks about the inspiration behind his sixty-six-day AT traverse, he calls upon a different quotation from George Mallory: "One must know the end to be convinced that one can win the end."

I know this is the third time Mallory's been mentioned in this chapter. And it's worth noting that no one really knows if this extraordinary British mountaineer ever reached Everest's summit, since he died before he ever made it back down. But he was as quotable as Yogi Berra, and I for one like to think he made it to the summit. I have no interest in being a tragic hero nor do I think any of the FKT athletes I know have a death wish. But the blinding drive to reach a fixed point on a map is a shared connection. There's something found in those final steps to the summit that can't be discovered anywhere else.

After setting a record, I was frequently asked if it was more a challenge of the body or of the mind. Or as one journalist put it succinctly, "Is it more physical or mental?"

It's hard to say. My answers tended to vacillate and contradict themselves.

Horton's response to the same question was concise, but no less confusing. He said, "Both."

The external challenges are going to be there—having twenty-five thousand feet of elevation change in a day, slogging through relentless thunderstorms, or trudging through hundred-degree heat and humidity. Even though I took sports psychology and had some tools to fall back on, at times it *still* seemed that I was playing a game I couldn't win, that I was fighting not one but two formidable opponents. The external challenges beat you till you're black and blue, then the internal ones chew you up and spit you out for good measure. It can be a vicious cycle, and sometimes both opponents are pummeling you so hard it's impossible to tell them apart. It's not always like that, but just as sure as you're going to face injuries on an FKT, you're going to face emotional doubts. And if you don't bring your A game both mentally and physically on an FKT attempt, it's highly unlikely that you will be successful.

The same way that athletes have different training regimens to get ready for a competition, others will approach obstacles with different mental strategies. David Horton and I both believe in the value of a higher power, particularly when you are in a weakened state.

Dr. Czech confirmed that "calling upon a transcendental purpose can be an important psychological skill when it comes to endurance."

David Horton found what he needed in his faith. Like Horton, I relied on my beliefs, but I also drew strength from my husband's love and the vitality of the forest. I'm not trying to sound overly religious, sappy, or new age but more than my legs, that's what got me to the end.

When I lost that curiosity to keep going and no longer cared what my best was, I stuck with it because I wanted to thank my husband for his support by persevering.

The couple that gave us premarital counseling told us it was important to "dream dreams" and support each other's goals. They mentioned things like signing up for a cooking class or traveling to far-off places. They did *not* give the example of trying to set an FKT on the Appalachian Trail. By all accounts, my dream was straight-up bat-shit crazy. But Brew supported me nonetheless.

As he was my primary crew person, I witnessed firsthand and was the beneficiary of all the selfless tasks he performed throughout the day. He believed in me, and I didn't want to let him down. Seeing him at each road crossing made me want to go back into the forest.

Conversely, the inspiration I felt from the forest helped me push on to the next road crossing. Sometimes, I would graze my fingertips against the corrugated bark of the hardwood trees I passed. Occasionally I would stop to catch my breath and lean against the soft, velvetlike moss that covered a glacier erratic. And I would draw strength from the fact that this giant boulder deposited millions of years ago by a receding ice flow served as my rest stop.

There was something about touching the forest, the tactile transfer of energy, that provided strength. Physically connecting with the environment, breathing in the thick sweetness of the evening air, it was as if my body absorbed some kind of all-natural, Appalachia-based electrolyte.

Every trail I've hiked has a different feel, a distinct aura. The Appalachian Trail emits wisdom. There is a palpable maturity that wafts through the ancient granite and the exposed, gnarled roots of the spruce trees. It's like the loving embrace of a wrinkled grandmother, and on several occasions, that enduring force gave me an energy I couldn't find within myself.

I also prayed a lot. On a long-distance hike of any sort, either you talk to God or you talk to yourself. I did a fair bit of both. I could tell myself till I was blue in the face that I was meant to be on that trail. But when I talked to God I was convinced I belonged.

Eric Liddell, the Olympic runner who was portrayed in the movie *Chariots of Fire*, famously said, "I feel like God made me for a purpose, but he also made me fast! And when I run I feel His pleasure." I started thinking that my ability to hike was a gift and a divine responsibility. The farther I walked, the weaker I felt, the more I relied on my faith, and the more I felt God's presence. The FKT shares similar traits with an ascetic fast, a solitary retreat, or native ritual rife with hallucinogens. When I walk through the forest I feel closer to my God. I'll never be able to offer a clear explanation for that. But I sure as heck won't let anybody explain it away, either.

Not everyone prays his or her way to the finish.

I might joke that Scott Williamson set an FKT for his cat, but he said, "I have never felt that I necessarily held to a transcendent or higher cause to keep me going through the rough times."

Still, he admits that there are times when something inexplicable happens in matters of endurance.

"I will say there have been times where I truly have no idea how I made it through the day, times when I felt there was just no way it was going to happen and somehow it did. When I am out there pushing myself, something *does* happen that allows me to do more than I can in my day-to-day life."

As for Warren, I once heard him give a ninety-minute presentation on his higher power from the worn wooden pews of a Methodist church in rural Appalachia. The setting belied Warren's lack of interest in organized religion of any sort. Instead, throughout his talk he referenced social change and the trail itself as his motivations for making forward progress.

He concluded the presentation by queuing up slides on his seventies-era projector and simultaneously pressing the play button on his boom box. The cassette tape had been fast-forwarded (because that's what you do with a cassette tape) to the beginning of Steve Winwood's 1986 hit "Higher Love." Warren tapped his foot along to the beat as Winwood sang. The song ended with Warren, in his matching tie-dyed ensemble of T-shirt *and* pants, twirling beneath the shots on the screen and waving his arms to the Chaka Khan refrain.

Like so many tie-dyed, twirling, boom-box-toting hippies of the twenty-first century, Warren found his deeper purpose in a higher love. Granted, most of those tie-dyed hippies probably leaned more toward Jerry Garcia than Steve Winwood. But the message of the music was the same. And like Scott Williamson's story of "The Gambler," Warren's dancing to the rhythms of "Higher Love" stuck with me for a long, *long* time.

When Dr. Czech and I discussed the significance of a transcendent cause on performance, he said, "A higher power is intrinsic to the individual and the best motivation is intrinsic because you can control it. And you can't control external factors."

Control is one of four building blocks for optimal performance as defined by practitioners of sports psychology. The "four Cs" are control, commitment, concentration, and confidence.

I like control and letting go of it is hard. (If anyone feels different, then I would like to get the number for her therapist.) When I couldn't affect my environment or circumstances on the trail, I seized the one thing I could control: my response. In other words, I couldn't change my reality but I could change how I thought about it.

I could curse the rain or I could splash in the puddles.

I could get frustrated at taking a wrong turn or I could appreciate seeing a different section of trail.

I could scream and cry as I hike through an overgrown patch of painful, stinging nettles or I could scream and cry and be grateful that the irritating burn caused by the plant fibers goes away after fifteen minutes and doesn't last all day.

Dr. Czech defines control as "staying in charge, no matter the situation. Despite the storms, roadblocks, and fire you are still in control of *you*." And in that sense, control is achievable and essential for an FKT athlete—or anyone, doing anything, ever.

Controlling your response is not a Jedi mind trick, it is a simple act of taking a deep breath and choosing how you will react to the information at hand. It offers a way to insert optimism, personal strength, and thoughtfulness into any situation.

For example, when my husband chews his food so loudly that I can hear him eating in another room, I can get frustrated and annoyed or I can simply remind myself—and Brew—how much I love him. And if this were a real scenario, I might even yell, "At least when I hear your chewing it lets me know you're alive."

Control is something we continually grasp for, and more often than not we come up empty-handed. But it is important to practice exerting what control we have and crafting careful responses, in light of the circumstances that surround us.

Getting involved with an FKT is like falling in love. There's the honeymoon phase in the beginning. It's romantic, you get chocolates and flowers, and you're blessed with beautiful sunsets and a sense of euphoria. But if the feeling of butterflies is all you've got, the relationship isn't going to last. At some point the requirement shifts from passion and planning to a monumental commitment. There are moments of exhilaration, but there are also times when it's an utter grind, and if you don't accept it as an undulating journey of highs and lows then it's not going to work in the long run.

Dr. Czech defines commitment as "the ability to never give up, the idea that you are all in."

I found that word "ability" interesting, because he could have said "the idea of never giving up" or "the desire to never give up." But ideas and desires don't convey talent or effort as the word "ability" does. We can't just want commitment; we have to work at it.

When I asked Dr. Czech about concentration, he brought up Joan of Arc. "She ran into battle when she was *seventeen*, leading a bunch of men. Literally leading them to fight. A general rebuffed her, claiming his men wouldn't follow her lead. Her response was, 'It doesn't matter whether you follow me or not. I'm not looking back.' Now *that's* concentration."

To me, Joan of Arc embodies not just concentration, but all four Cs. Born as a fifteenth-century French peasant girl, she became a teenage war hero and a religious martyr. She only lived nineteen years, but her commitment, confidence, and control have made her a mainstream figure for the past six hundred years, and a canonized saint, but if Dr. Czech wants to list her under concentration I can roll with that.

I knew that trying to set a trail record would take a hefty dose of concentration. What I didn't realize is the toll that it would take. On one hand, I loved being single-focused for an extended period. On the other hand, there were other things that I wanted to give my attention to. But I knew that I couldn't shift my focus and still be successful.

One of my very close friends who had dealt with fertility issues suffered a miscarriage when I was going for the record. It was heartbreaking not to be there for her. I spent several hours hiking with tears streaming down my face. When I made it to the next road crossing, Brew asked me what had taken so long. My pace had dropped, I felt dehydrated and emotionally drained.

Brew assured me that my dear friend would want me to keep hiking—I knew that's what she wanted. She almost didn't tell me about the miscarriage because she didn't want to distract me from the record. The fact that she considered a devastating loss to be a distraction, the fact that it was a distraction, made me feel like a shitty friend. But I knew that I needed to put it behind me and kept hiking. That's the problem with setting a record. Holding that type of concentration for forty-six days is impressive, but it's not always good.

I'm glad that I no longer have to be single-focused for weeks at a time, but I think the pendulum might have swung too far the other way. Having a young child, and owning a smartphone, have made it to where I can't make a cup of coffee without checking the weather forecast, replying to a text, packing my daughter's lunch for day care, and then going into the bathroom to help her "wipe."

Instead of taking five minutes to smell the aroma of my dark roast and watch steaming brown liquid fill my mug, I push the brew button and then walk away to address multiple random needs. Sometime midmorning, I come back to collect my cold drink and then chug it to medicate my caffeine headache, which is what reminded me that I forgot my coffee in the first place.

I might not sign up for another task as ambitious and all-consuming as a trail record, but holding my concentration for forty-six days reminds me that I can still do small things well. I can put my cell phone down, I can ask my daughter to wait patiently or empower her to handle bathroom matters without help, and I can focus a few minutes of my day on making a hot beverage.

One small action, a few minutes devoted to single-mindedness, has the ability to make the whole day better—especially if it involves coffee.

To my surprise, when I asked Dr. Czech about the idea of confidence, he started talking about failure. "Everyone's going to fail once in a while. But you still have to believe that you can accomplish your goal. There's no getting down in the mouth. You tell yourself tomorrow's going to be a better day and you keep going." I immediately thought of Scott Williamson, the person who has failed more and accomplished more than any other hiker I know. Scott makes failure look easy, and I mean that as a compliment.

Most FKTers have a handful of failed attempts that surround their accomplishments. That's just the way it goes when you're up against so many variables.

Warren Doyle was successful when he went after the record in 1973. But after John Avery lowered his mark, Warren went back to try to reclaim the title. Less than a week into his hike, he was a full two days ahead of his previous time and almost that far ahead of John's itinerary, too.

But as he neared Stecoah Gap in North Carolina, he felt a sharp pain below his foot socket. He looked down to see if a snake had bitten through his shoe, but the ground was still. He decided to keep moving, but as he continued down the trail, he felt an incendiary pain shoot up his right leg.

"It was almost like a chemical reaction," he told me. "It traveled up the right side of my body, swirled around my skull, then went down the left side. Within minutes the skin behind my knees and opposite my elbows was purple. I got to the road at the gap and sat down to take off my shoe."

He didn't find a bee or any indication that he'd been stung or bitten, but he entire foot was swollen and blue. He flagged the next car that came around the turn and hitched a ride to nearby Robbinsville.

"When I arrived at the clinic," he said, "I felt like I was going to black out. I walked up to the desk and there wasn't anyone there so I went into the back looking for help. Eventually I found a nurse, and I knew I was in trouble when I saw her reaction. I was on the verge of going into anaphylactic shock. I guess at that point my lips were blue and swollen. They immediately gave me an injection, but after thirty minutes I still hadn't come out of it so they gave me another round of epinephrine."

Later that morning, when he was no longer purple and blue from head to toe, Warren debated returning to the trail. He hobbled over to the nurses' station and asked what his chances of dying would have been if he hadn't have made it to the clinic. "Fifty percent," she said matter-of-factly. Warren had used up his luck; he decided to go home.

David Horton isn't used to failure. He's won dozens of races, inspired hundreds if not thousands of East Coast runners, and set new FKTs on both the AT and the PCT his first time around. Then in 2008 he went out to the Rockies and the Continental Divide Trail in an effort to become the first person to set an FKT on the three biggest trails in the United States, the "Triple Crown" of hiking. He lasted a day.

"I've been through the Mojave desert a few times," he said. "It's not that bad. The Chihuahuan desert, now *that's* bad. When you start at the border, there are just these two pieces of barbed wire that separate the United States from Mexico. I didn't see any border patrol. I guess they decided they don't need to patrol that section because if you cross over, you'll probably die in the desert anyway. I made it thirty or thirty-five miles before I got lost and dehydrated.

"I was supposed to see my crew at some point in the middle of the day and we never connected. I'd run out of water and I only had a handful of food. When I stopped to rest at a cattle trough, my watch said it was 110 degrees.

"As soon as I sat down my entire body started cramping—my calves, quads, hamstrings, everything. I couldn't move and I didn't know which direction to go. I said, 'Lord, this is stupid.' I knew it was going to be a long time before anyone would find me out there in the middle of nowhere.

"Finally, I decided I had to drink. So I dipped my bottle under the green scum that lined the top of the trough. I had a few sips of brown water and finished my food. Then I drank some more. I started to feel a little bit better and decided I had to keep moving. I pointed my compass north and followed it to the next road. I had to guess whether to go right or left, but I chose the right direction and found my crew. I slept a few hours, then tried to keep going, but they said, 'You can't do that.' And I thought, yeah, I can't do that. So it ended."

"How did you feel?" I asked. I know Horton, and I knew what he'd say but I asked him anyway.

"Horrible," he said. "Worthless. I hate failing. I feel like such a fraud and a fake." Then he smiled and shrugged.

It's remarkable—and a little disconcerting—that a man who has achieved so much can get so demoralized by having to admit defeat. I guess that's the insecurity talking.

If David had "failed" as many times as Scott Williamson had on long-distance trails, he might not be able to look himself in the mirror. Fortunately, Scott has a more forgiving opinion of himself and his erratic track record.

"I've quit several FKT attempts," he said, "more than I've finished successfully, in fact. When I've had to bail, I've generally not felt that bad about it, because every time I've quit, I've known in my heart with 100 percent certainty that there was no way I could continue onward." (By Warren's measure Scott didn't quit; he stopped.)

"Sure, it's a letdown. It always is. But it's not as bad as you would think, because as soon as it's happened, I'm already trying to learn what I can from it to improve on the next one, which I'll already be planning before I get off the trail."

"If you never fail then you haven't set your goals high enough." That's what my summer camp director told us in the dining hall one morning. He was a remarkable man and I admired him greatly, so I took in everything he ever said. But that thought has stuck with me more than all of his other truisms combined.

One of the main reasons I decided to try for the Appalachian Trail record was that I'd never started a thru hike and not finished or set a mileage or time goal I didn't meet. If I wanted to find my best, I had to be willing to fail. And I'm not talking a "moral victory" kind of failure. I'm talking about the epic "crash and burn" kind.

I did have to wrestle the possibility of disappointment to the ground before I ever got going.

The biggest hurdle for me wasn't the hundred-mile training weeks or the logistics of planning a forty-six-day adventure; it was the fear of failure. I didn't want to look bad in front of an audience, even if the "audience" was only friends and family and a handful of admirers online.

One of the most empowering aspects of the journey was that I was forced to overcome my personal vanity before stepping on the trail. This wasn't about how I looked; it was about what I could do. As Warren said about his record, "My one motivation in attempting the record was to rediscover myself under the judgment of the trail rather than society." Ultimately, I had to let go of public perception to hold on to a dream, and doing that was one of the most empowering aspects of the journey.

I can understand how some people might view an FKT as narcissistic, or, as Nancy Horton said, "based on ego." But it cuts both ways. Subjecting yourself to the possibility of failure—especially when you're in the public eye—takes some cojones, or in my case blatant nerve. Vulnerability isn't just a willingness to admit your weakness; it's also the ability to risk your strengths and talents without the promise of success. I chose to put my vulnerability above my social image. I was going to either fail or succeed. But I sure as hell wasn't going to be complacent.

My camp director's logic suggests that because I didn't fail on my record attempt there is still room for improvement. And perhaps that is true, but it's worth pointing out that I felt as if I failed over and over again throughout the hike. There were stretches where I got lost, days when I didn't reach my mileage goals, and a handful of times in the first few weeks when I flat-out hit the wall. I spent most of the summer thinking I wouldn't be able to set the record. But I continued anyway.

My reward was *more* than the answer I found on that final mountain. It was also the freedom I'd felt when I shoved off of that very first summit, staring the distinct possibility of public failure and humiliation in the face and saying, "Screw it. I'm gonna try anyway." Coming to terms with the possibility of not setting the record and going after it anyway was every bit as empowering as a successful finish.

At this point, my work and family prevent me from setting my FKT goals any higher. But the truth is I don't want to go after any more trail records. What I want is to continue to take risks and put myself out there. It might be in relationships at work, or even through a hobby, but I want to always be in a position where I might fail.

I have great admiration for my husband, because he has taken up singing, songwriting, and playing the guitar in his late thirties. Nearly every night after we put our daughter to sleep he practices strumming, finger picking, and then picks up his pen and works on a song. Every few weeks, he goes to open mic nights, takes his slot amid lifelong musicians, and performs a set of original songs for strangers. Brew's willingness to expand his artistry and expose his talent along with his flaws is attractive, and it challenges me to hold on to my dreams and pursue new goals. We all need loved ones who take risks and hold us accountable to growth. Stagnation and adventure are both infectious.

My beloved camp director who encouraged me to set high goals also taught me how to start each day on a positive note. At the end of breakfast each morning he would lead us in a campwide refrain. And, in unison, four hundred girls and young women shouted, "It's a great day and I feel terrific." I was all in, and I learned that when you start the morning on a positive note and state your desired intentions for the day, you tend to be a happier and more productive person.

As an adult, I still start my day by speaking my intentions into the universe, however much my chorus has changed over time. Now I stumble into the bathroom, put my palms on the vanity, stare up at the mirror, and ask myself, "What can I fail at today?" It's not self-deprecating; it's invigorating.

Life feels a whole lot more worth living when you have something to lose. Holding myself accountable to risk is far more refreshing than splashing cold water on my face. But that comes next. (Risk tolerance doesn't do much for the drool streak on your cheek or dark circles under your eyes.) Then, the coffee.

I remember Dr. Czech repeating the definition of one very important term almost every time our sports psychology class met. The term was "mental toughness."

"Mental toughness," he'd say, "is the ability to focus, to rebound from failure, to cope with pressure, and to persist in the face of adversity. It is," and here he'd pause for dramatic effect, "the *essence* of sports psychology."

I didn't know it then, but Dr. Czech was actively preparing me for tackling trail records . . . and parenting . . . and running a small business.

Years later I asked him if there was any difference between the mental toughness of an endurance athlete and that of, say, a baseball player or a gymnast or sprinter.

"In a lot of ways, it's the same," he said. "The mental toughness you've developed—the resiliency, the vigor, the focus, goal setting, self-confidence, regulating stress—all of those are skills that you'd use in every sport. The difference with what you do is that you have to repeat those skills over and over and over again without a break."

"So when you think about the takeaways and applying sports to life, is there any benefit in opting for an endurance sport? I mean, is there a good reason to choose suffering?"

My wise old professor just laughed. "So you're trying to justify the hurt, huh?"

He paused for a second, then said, "Listen, sports psychology is the study of the brain's impact on performance. But it also looks at how performance affects the brain. The skills that you use are all skills that you can use in everyday life. They're skills you transfer to work, your family, *any* type of performance. I have to assume that the longevity of the trail helps you not only to become mentally tough but to *stay* mentally tough. And that's a pretty valuable life skill."

Mental toughness matters regardless of the endeavor. And, ultimately, I think that's the "why." That is the answer when people want to know the common motivation behind endurance athletes. It's a means to explore, expand, and extend our mental toughness. We need people who can demonstrate the physical capacity of the human body. But more than that, we need examples of how the brain can cope with suffering, overcome failures, and continue to persevere. That is the larger value of an FKT; that is why these pursuits matter.

CHAPTER SIX

An Unapologetic American Male

"Drink some water. Go for a run. Have an attitude adjustment
and stop thinking so god damn much."

—Andrew Thompson

Andrew Thompson is a twenty-first-century cowboy. He doesn't ride horses or drive cattle, but he is ruggedly handsome, he never passes up a strong drink or a chance to sleep under the stars, and he *always* speaks his mind. It can be difficult to describe Andrew's physique and charisma without sounding as if you have a thing for him. But it can be just as challenging to portray his confidence without making him out to be a cocky bastard.

Andrew's personality is cut from the same cloth as that of the iconic Western film star Marion Michael Morrison, otherwise known as John Wayne. They share a personality capable of owning their faults, parading their strengths, and never seeing a need to separate the two.

Morrison said, "Each of us is a mixture of some good and some not so good qualities. In considering one's fellow man it's important to remember the good things. . . . We should refrain from making judgments just because a fella happens to be a dirty, rotten SOB."

The difference between John Wayne and Andrew Thompson when compared to almost everyone else is that each would admit to being a dirty rotten SOB with a smile on his face. The rest of us are too prideful or ashamed to admit it.

When I first met Andrew I wasn't interested in trail records and I didn't know what the initials FKT meant.

We were headed in opposite directions. I was three hundred miles from the finish of my first thru hike; Andrew was three hundred miles into his AT record attempt. I had been on the trail four months; Andrew had been out there for ten days. I only had 15 percent of the footpath left to hike, compared to Andrew's 85 percent. And yet when I saw him, I was far more confident in his chance of finishing than in my own. To see Andrew in action is to know he *owned* the fastest known time (I'm a quick learner), even before he actually set it.

I'm not short, but he towered over me. When we crossed paths, he was going uphill and I was descending. Still, my gait needed to double in order to match his footprints. His build was so strong, his shoulders so broad, that he seemed to create a draft that forced the gaunt thru hikers ahead of me off the trail in his wake.

But more than anything it was his smile, his relaxed nature, and the banter he shared with his trail companion—an only slightly shorter version of himself—that convinced me Andrew was destined for the record. We were on Mount Washington, one of the most unforgiving peaks in the world and arguably the toughest climb on the entire Appalachian Trail, but Andrew and his friend made everything about the outing seem easy and lighthearted.

When I eventually caught up with the three male thru hikers who were ahead of me on the descent, they were comparing notes and agreeing that this most conspicuous figure, the one with the intimidating stride and raucous laugh, had come across as a pompous jackass. But I was mesmerized.

Andrew Thompson reached Springer Mountain a few weeks after I summited Katahdin. He had set a new FKT. There was never any doubt he would.

But what I didn't realize then and what I wouldn't learn until years later was that the striking, self-assured young man on Mount Washington was not on his first Appalachian Trail record attempt. It was his fourth try. I also didn't know that he had spent most of his twenties healing from a legalistic religious upbringing or that he had recently been divorced. And I didn't learn about the grueling nine-day journey that preceded his hike up Mount Washington until nearly a decade later.

It turns out I was wrong; nothing about his hike up Mount Washington was easy. He just made it look that way. The man I observed bounding up the mountain wasn't hiding or running from the hardships he'd faced; he was happily embracing the struggle.

There is a conflicting warmth and harshness to Andrew Thompson's personality. It is mirrored in his New Hampshire farmstead. On the surface its setting—with the stocked trout pond and acres of rolling countryside—is picturesque and inviting. But the reality is that it demands countless hours of backbreaking labor—keeping up the house, weeding the vegetable garden, caring for hogs in the barn, cutting and culling fallen timber, and boiling maple syrup in the sugar shack.

When I arrived at the farmhouse, located in one of the Granite State's rural upper valleys, Andrew's two thigh-high, tanned-skin, rambunctious boys greeted me. Aged four and two, the boys were happily wandering back and forth between the house and backyard, either harassing the family's border collie or being herded by it.

When I walked into the craftsman-style house, Andrew's wife, Bethany, greeted me and took a break from cooking supper for the boys to offer me a comfortable chair and a glass of ice water. At first glance, Bethany's petite build and graceful, hospitable demeanor make her seem mild and unassuming. But it didn't take long for her intelligence and strength to be laid bare by a stream of incisive questions and the tasks she made quick work of while alternating kids on and off her hip.

After I had visited with Bethany for a half hour, trying not to be collateral damage amid the whirlwind of energy and flying toys created by two young boys, Andrew pushed through the front door, drenched in sweat from his latest athletic conquest, leaving a trail of salt water behind him on the cold tile floor. He greeted me with a broad grin and an engulfing hug that left a wet imprint on my clean clothes. He then excused himself for a quick shower, returning in a pair of faded blue jeans loosely held to his hips by a leather belt. In true Andrew fashion, he had disregarded the need for a shirt.

After affectionately kissing his family good night, Andrew grabbed a can of beer from the fridge, popped the top, and motioned for me to follow him outside, where we jumped into his red, well-worn pickup and peeled out for a nearby trailhead.

With the windows rolled down, Andrew had one hand on the clutch and the other on his beer. He kept the truck in its lane with his legs and the occasional and brief correction from his fingertips. With a smirk on his face and the wind blowing through his hair, he let out an uproarious laugh before launching into a profanity-laced tirade against religion, knowing full well that our theological stances are opposed. I couldn't help but smile and laugh as Andrew slammed my theological worldview. I wouldn't expect anything less from him. His favorite form of conversation is good-natured controversy.

When we arrived at the trailhead, Andrew dropped his empty beer can on the truck's floorboard, changed into shorts and a T-shirt, grabbed a flashlight, and then let me take the lead as we began hiking through the cool air of a New England summer's eve.

Andrew followed my footsteps as we traveled up the gently graded path to the top of Mount Tom in Woodstock, Vermont. The conversation ranged from his sheltered, rigid upbringing—which contextualized his cynical views on religion—to a discussion of trail records and endurance athletes. Andrew is unapologetic in his opinions and life choices, as well as the descriptors he uses for close friends and complete strangers. As we discussed trail records, Andrew was quick to comment on a list of highly revered athletes and their accomplishments. He painted colorful pictures of men and women whom I had read about in black and white.

When we started talking about trends that link endurance

athletes, I looked back at him and asked, "Do you think you struggle with insecurity?"

"No," he said. Then he thought about it a second longer. "Fuck no."

In a way, Andrew's entire life has been defined by breaking the rules. Rules saturated his childhood. He was raised with stringent guidelines that made him feel that he was bound to fail. As the son of an evangelical preacher in a small New England town, he was expected to uphold the family's image and doctrine every minute of every day. His life was a prison of organized religion.

Andrew's father, Chip, served as the senior pastor at New England Bible Church in Andover, Massachusetts; however, he was not always a religious fanatic nor was he raised in a Christian home. "But he was intense and passionate, like me," Andrew said. "He was completely committed to whatever he was doing."

As a free-wheeling twenty-year-old living in California, Chip funneled his energy into surfing. "He was really good," Andrew claims. "He traveled all over for surfing competitions." Then one day on the beach in Santa Cruz, Chip met a Czechoslovakian who was proselytizing Jesus to the unsaved surfers. "I'm not sure what the hell that man said but it must have been pretty convincing."

So Chip traded in his surfboard for a Bible and left behind the rolling waters of the Southern California coast for the "living waters" of evangelical Christianity. He traveled across country with his young wife, Joan, to attend Pensacola Christian College in Florida, a school where biology classes taught that the world was created less than ten thousand years ago in six twenty-four-hour cycles.

Chip was a student there when his son was born. Then, when Andrew was five years old, his family moved to Massachusetts so that Chip could start a church to reach the nonbelievers in New England, the Yankee heathens. (And the southerner in me can't help but smile at that.)

Andrew was enrolled in kindergarten at a small Christian school just over the Massachusetts state line in New Hampshire. He stayed there for the next twelve years. "It was probably the worst school in the state," Andrew recalls. "My parents paid money for me to attend the worst school in New Hampshire because they thought I should have a Christian education. Every day at school there was chapel or Bible class. Even regular classes had to begin with prayer or some kind of devotional. Everything had to be justified. Before *basketball practice*, the coach had to find some obscure Bible reference to set the tone and justify what we were doing."

At home his father's work commitments dictated Andrew's schedule. He was expected to be at church every Sunday morning, Sunday evening, and Wednesday night. He frequented prayer meetings and revivals and was expected to help entertain a constant stream of visiting missionaries and their children.

Andrew's father's strict beliefs bled into his child rearing. Andrew didn't have choices to make; he had expectations to meet. And the expectations were severe.

"And your mom just went along with what your dad wanted?" I asked.

"Well, they're divorced now," Andrew said with a laugh. "So not always. But when I was growing up she backed my dad. I guess that was her role as a good preacher's wife.

"This will give you an idea of the home I grew up in: One time when I was thirteen or fourteen, I traded watches with a girl at school for a day. I came home wearing her Timex and my parents flipped out. They thought it was 'lustful and covetous' or some shit like that. They demanded that I hand over the watch immediately and then they grounded me. They grounded me for wearing some girl's watch!"

I listened and shook my head in disbelief. I had grown up in the Bible Belt and had attended a Baptist college in Alabama, and I had never met anyone who had been more abused by doctrine than Andrew. That's the funny thing about religion—one person's liberation is another person's hell.

It comes as no surprise that Andrew longed for an escape. And the only place he felt free was outside his house, outside his school, outside his father's church. The only place he felt free was outside.

"When I was outside I could come and go as I pleased," he said. "It gave me something I needed. I genuinely fell in love with the outdoors."

"So you were always into it?" I asked.

"Yeah, I was always into it. I've always been fascinated with streams, rocks, plants, flowers, birds, trees, and different ecosystems. And I could do what I *wanted* out there. I could throw my baseball glove and fishing pole on my back and go ten miles away from home with no cell phone. That was my adventure."

Despite all the organized religion in his life, Andrew found his salvation in the forest.

When he graduated from high school, Andrew's parents told him he would attend Pensacola Christian College in Florida.

"Did your parents pay for it?" I asked.

"No!" he said. "*I* paid for it. I am still paying for a Christian education that I didn't want. I got down there and a barbed-wire fence surrounded the school. And the barbed wire was facing in! Do you understand what I am saying?

"I remember I went to my RA (residential advisor) and said, 'Why is the barbed wire around the campus facing in? Shouldn't it be facing out?' And, he looked at me and said, 'Whatever, it's just barbed wire.'

"Can you believe that?! 'It's just barbed wire.' That is literally what the guy said."

First-year students weren't allowed to leave campus, but Andrew found a way to sneak out and go for runs. He wasn't a runner in high school; he had always played team sports. But in Pensacola he needed an outlet, an escape, so he took to running. Within eight months, Andrew managed to run a mile in under five minutes and finish his first marathon. But he never felt that he was running fast enough or far enough to escape.

After his first year at Pensacola Christian College, Andrew returned to New Hampshire for the summer and informed his parents that, as he put it, "he was never, ever, going back to jail." He refused to return to Pensacola and he quit going to church.

"That's when Sundays went from being my least favorite day of the week to my favorite day of the week," he said. "Every weekend I would head up to the White Mountains in New Hampshire to climb four-thousand-foot peaks."

Because Andrew refused to return to Florida, his parents presented him with a list of more liberal Christian universities to choose from for the fall semester. Liberal was a relative term. His ultimate choice was Liberty University in Lynchburg, Virginia. It was the same Liberty University that had been founded by conservative televangelist Jerry Falwell, the same university that imposed a campuswide curfew, did not allow female students to wear shorts to class, and forbade members of the opposite sex from spending time alone together in unlit areas after dark. Most important, though, it was the same Liberty University where David Horton served as professor of exercise science.

For Andrew, Liberty lived up to its name. Compared to Pensacola Christian College, it was freedom. Instead of barbed wire surrounding the campus, there were dozens of miles of single track that spread deep into the forest, away from the academic buildings and the chapel. Andrew quickly began exploring the terrain. He was making new friends, trying new things, and starting to have a more typical college experience.

What wasn't typical for a nineteen-year-old was toeing the line at a fifty-mile ultramarathon. Andrew read about the fifty-mile Mountain Masochist Trail Run near Lynchburg in *UltraRunning* magazine. He registered for the race before he arrived on campus; it was one of the reasons he decided to go to Liberty.

The Masochist was founded by David Horton in 1983. Since then, the race has been a proving ground for trail runners across the Southeast. On a brisk day in early November, after ten hours and twenty-six minutes running through the mountains, Andrew felt as if he had been set free. He was greeted at the finish with the sound of a bullhorn and a huge hug; he was greeted by a man who would help him go even farther.

From that point forward, Andrew spent every Saturday—often morning, noon, and night—running with David Horton and a dedicated group of Lynchburg ultrarunners.

He grilled Horton for hours and miles on end and asked him to describe his adventures, particularly the AT record. Andrew said, "Every time we were out there I was picking his brain."

He listened to Horton wax eloquent about race strategy and made mental notes as The Runner described each of the ultras he had completed. Andrew didn't talk as much as Horton—nobody does—but he did quietly start to formulate and execute his own adventures. Over the next two and a half years, he participated in several dozen ultramarathons, finishing faster and placing higher as time wore on.

To hear Andrew talk about this seminal period of his life, one would think running was paramount. But there were other developments.

At the age of twenty-one, Andrew Thompson got married.

"You mention that like it was a nonevent," I said.

"It *was* a nonevent. It was just an absurd concept for two people who were that young and that indoctrinated to get married. Our parents pushed us into it. Are we really assuming that a twenty-one-year-old male didn't want to have sex? Or live with my girlfriend? With my background, there was only one way to make that happen. We got married so we could do the things that normal couples do. We got married so we could have sex."

"That's romantic," I said with a smirk.

Andrew laughed.

"I'm not trying to justify it," he said. "It is what it is."

Being married did not tie Andrew down.

He had spent the last two and a half years learning about endurance at the feet of David Horton and now he wanted to take down The Runner's FKT.

"How did Horton take it when you told him you were going after his record?"

"I didn't tell him," Andrew said.

"You didn't tell him?"

Andrew laughed. "No, but he found out anyway. He came to my room the week I was getting ready to leave and confronted me."

"Was he more upset that you were going after his record or that you didn't tell him about it?"

"I don't know. Both."

The fact that he said both made me laugh. It was a Hortonism. The professor's favorite response to a difficult either-or question.

"Did he give you any advice?"

"He had been giving me advice without knowing it for the past two years."

Andrew might not have shared his intentions, but if imitation is the highest form of flattery, then Andrew's record attempt demonstrated high esteem for his mentor. Not only did Andrew set out to claim Horton's record, he copied nearly every detail of it. He started at Springer Mountain, Georgia, on the same *date* that Horton began. Andrew then followed Horton's exact itinerary, mile for mile, day by day.

From a strategic standpoint, Andrew's plan was commendable. Horton's well-publicized schedule provided a blueprint for the record. By matching Horton's numbers each day, Andrew could put forth the minimum output required to stay within reach of the fastest known time before surpassing Horton's mileage the last day or two of the run.

The only problem with his strategy was that there was very little margin for error. It started to rain when Andrew got to Connecticut, and the deluge continued for seven straight days. Andrew persisted through Massachusetts and into the Green Mountains of Vermont. There he started to fall off pace, unable to match Horton's miles through what he describes as "life-sucking mud."

In the early weeks of summer, Vermont—otherwise known as Vermud—is filled with a soft wet tread that will suction off your shoe. The locals call it "mud season." Trying to hike through it is comparable to trudging through ankle-deep snow or wading against the current of a river. It turns walking into a resistance sport. Your pace slows, your feet sink into the ground, and before you know it you are hopping backward on one foot to pull your sneaker out of what looks like brownie batter.

Andrew had made it through twelve states; he only had two left to go. But after running, hiking, and trudging through the rain and mud for a week, he quit.

Andrew went back to Lynchburg, back to his wife, back to his job at Outback Steakhouse, and back to running with Horton every Saturday. Andrew's relationship with Horton was relatively unaffected after his failed record attempt. Imitation is a high form of flattery, but imitation that results in failure is the ultimate ego stroke.

There was one big change the following fall; Andrew did not return to Liberty for the upcoming semester. He was twenty-one years old, a legal adult, and he was ready for something other than a Christian education. He enrolled in a nearby liberal arts college and continued working toward his degree.

"It took a while to graduate," he admitted. "I floated through my twenties. I'd run and work and go to school on and off. There wasn't any rhyme or reason to it. But I always knew I'd go back to the trail."

Andrew did not return to the trail, though, until the record had been lowered substantially.

In 1999, Pete Palmer, a postal worker from Connecticut, came to the AT and lowered the record from Horton's fifty-two days to forty-eight. Bringing it below the half-century mark and reducing the elapsed time by three and a half days was a monumental feat, and all the credit in the world should be—and was—directed at Pete and his crew.

But when you look at his record, one statistic that is arguably as shocking as his daily miles is the fact that he spent forty-eight days on the trail and got only *one day* of rain. He hiked through oppressive heat and humidity but did not have constant afternoon thundershowers like David Horton and he wasn't hit with a nor'easter in Vermont like Andrew. Record setters go after the same mark but they never experience the same trail.

In 2001, three years after his first record attempt, Andrew returned to the trail to challenge Pete's record. He was still self-funded through his job at Outback, he was still working toward a degree, he was still married, although this year he decided that no women—wives or girlfriends—were allowed to be a part of the crew during the record attempt. "It was a boys' trip," he said. "I didn't want any distractions." He needed to concentrate.

The fastest known time was three and a half days shorter than it had been on Andrew's first attempt and his run would be more challenging because of it. But when he got on the trail in Georgia that May, he was sure that he would set the record.

This time he didn't get stuck in the mud; he made it through thirteen states and arrived at the base of the Presidential Range in New Hampshire on July 2, right on schedule. Then he started climbing up the slopes of Mount Washington with his crew chief and best friend, J.B.

The wind picked up, the clouds rolled in, and the temperature dropped precipitously. When Andrew and J.B. left the tree line, the weather transitioned from uncomfortable to life threatening. By the time they reached the rock-strewn ridgeline, fragile alpine plants were coated in several inches of rime ice and a smattering of hoar frost was lining their nostrils, lips, and eyelids. The wind was so strong that when they looked up to discern the course of the trail, their eyes filled with tears and their vision was blurred. It took every ounce of energy and resolve to force one foot ahead of the other.

When they reached the sanctuary of an Appalachian Mountain Club hut one and a half miles below the summit of Mount Washington, Andrew wasn't thinking about the record; he was thinking about how lucky they were to be alive. As he was sitting in the dining area at Lake of the Clouds Hut, trying to warm up with a lukewarm cup of coffee, a report came from the summit that wind speeds had reached eighty miles per hour and the wind chill had come in at negative twenty-one.

Andrew stood up and walked over to the coffee pot for a refill. His second AT record attempt was over. He would leave the hut and head home as soon as the weather allowed it. But you can't loiter at Lake of the Clouds for free—not even in a winter storm. So, adding insult to injury, Andrew agreed to a work-for-stay arrangement.

He spent the first few hours after his failed record attempt up to his elbows in dish soap, with J.B. by his side, scrubbing pots and pans for the privilege of taking a nap in the dank basement.

After he failed the second time, one might wonder if Andrew was a victim of bad luck or bad strategy. He never left himself any margin for error.

From the sidelines, I think Andrew could have made it through the mud in Vermont and still set the record. But he was young and his mental toughness wasn't where it needed to be.

Not pushing through the winter storm on Mount Washington was the right decision, the only decision. But if he had built a slight cushion to account for bad weather, he might have come home with the record.

Perhaps if he had started with more money, he could have built that lead. Instead, he'd started with a meager six hundred dollars in his pack and had relied on the frugality of his crew and the help of strangers to sustain the journey. You can't buy a trail record, but trying to be successful on a shoestring budget can negatively affect team morale.

I admit, it is always easier to be a commentator than the fighter in the ring. And while it is possible to critique his strategy and frugality, I'd be hard pressed to assert that Andrew could have had a better man in his corner.

From my own experience, I've come to believe that the task—the punishment—of lending emotional and logistical support to an exhausted, often irrational endurance athlete over the course of several weeks should be reserved for a close relative, a spouse, or a paid support person. The role should fall only on someone whose commitment to stay by your side is bound by blood or an oath or at the very least a payment schedule. The thought of having a close friend crew an FKT seems disastrous. But not for Andrew.

On his first go, Andrew's best friend from Lynchburg, J.B.—or "Jonboy"—crewed him into Vermont. Andrew occasionally had help from family members on his first hike. And he enlisted the services of another close friend to assist Jonboy on the second. But ultimately it was J.B. who gave up his summers to live on a shoestring budget, sleep in the bed of a Toyota Tacoma, and absorb the brunt of his friend's athletically induced hysteria—to *almost* set the record . . . twice.

When I first met Andrew and witnessed him muscling his way toward the Mount Washington summit, it was J.B. who was by his side. They were both physical specimens: tan, fit, and full of bravado. At the time I wondered if they were brothers. My assumption wasn't far off.

J.B. was also the first to volunteer when Andrew was ready to go back to the Appalachian Trail for a third try.

After spending time with Horton and Scott—and based on my own experience—I knew that a supportive spouse held just as much ownership of an FKT as his or her hiking-running counterpart. Regardless of whether a loved one is waiting at home alone, or schlepping gear and snacks to the next road crossing, there are sacrifices that are made in a marriage when the husband or wife sets an FKT.

What Andrew and J.B. made me realize is that the emotional support needed for endurance doesn't have to come from a spouse, but it's got to come from somewhere. Record setters are relational. Yes, a lot of us are introverts—not Andrew Thompson, mind you—but we all have identified certain people in our lives who can get us where we want to go and make the journey more pleasant.

FKT athletes don't just appreciate our close friends and family; we depend on them. When you look at the FKT proboards, you see the daily miles, but you don't see the spouse who steps into the role of single parent and sole provider so the other person can live his or her dream. When *Backpacker* magazine publishes a story about the next record setter, it focuses on the athlete, not the crew person who located a rural Laundromat to wash mildewed hiker clothes before rushing back to the trail to mix electrolyte drinks and cook dinner for someone who was going to stumble out of the woods in a bad mood.

When it comes to perseverance, you can last longer, cope better, and push farther when you have help. Outstanding feats of endurance require outstanding support.

Four years after being forced off Mount Washington in a snowstorm, Andrew was ready for another go at the record. His support crew was the same, but almost everything else looked different. He was recently divorced. Now he was dating his high school crush, Bethany. He was once again thinking about marriage, but this time he was willing to wait—at least to get married. "I always wanted to go out with her," he said. "But she was the type of girl that was always in a relationship. When I finally got my chance, I didn't want to blow it."

After eight years, he had finally finished his undergraduate degree and promptly left Lynchburg for New Hampshire. Once back in New

England, he started researching continuing-ed certifications in the medical field. He also began surfing—a lot. Three decades after his father rode a wave onto a beach in Southern California and found Jesus at the hands of an evangelical Czechoslovakian, Andrew started running into the icy New England waters trying to catch a break.

His natural athleticism, combined with a disciplined training regimen and a relentless willingness to endure cold water and crashing waves, helped him win his first surfing competition in the spring of 2005. At the same time, his physique and confident glare landed him on the cover of the *New York Times Magazine* with a longboard in hand.

He was no longer floating through his twenties. Now he was catching the current and riding the wave.

When Andrew set out on his third Appalachian Trail record attempt, he ascended Katahdin wearing a brown Eastern Surfing Association trucker hat. Besides being a trucker hat kind of guy, Andrew loved that his headwear didn't have anything to do with hiking or trail running or a stale energy bar sponsor. He wasn't trying to play the role of a record setter. This time he came to the trail with a greater sense of who he was and what he could do. He was ready to claim his identity—and the trail record.

Andrew decided to begin his journey in Maine, not in Georgia like David, Pete, or the record setters of the past. And this time he didn't carry anyone else's itinerary in his back pocket.

When comparing the trail conditions he'd had on his two attempts to the less than one day of rain Pete Palmer experienced, Andrew could easily have assumed that fate—or perhaps God—was against him. He could have been despondent; he could have been indignant. Instead, Andrew was motivated.

In many ways, Pete Palmer's setting the record was the best thing that could have happened to Andrew, because when a postal worker from Connecticut broke David Horton's time, it humanized the record and it demystified the endeavor.

The record was no longer held by a trail-running legend who had been Andrew's mentor and training partner. Now, in his mind, there wasn't just one direction and one itinerary to follow when attempting to make the fastest known time. And now Andrew didn't just think that he might barely be able to surpass someone else's mark; for the first time since setting foot on the trail, he wasn't trying to beat David. For the first time, he was out there because he wanted to discover what he could do.

Then, three days into his third attempt, Andrew quit.

When you don't follow a blueprint, you're more likely to access opportunity—and encounter misfortune. Andrew had started too soon. He left Katahdin on May 15 and quickly discovered that there was still snow on the ground above twenty-five hundred feet. It wasn't much better *below* twenty-five hundred feet, where the trail was a creek, the creeks were swollen rivers, and the clouds of blackflies and mosquitoes on the damp forest floor were cause for insanity.

The third time was *not* the charm, and any reasonable person might assume that after three strikes, one might become discouraged if not despondent. Andrew simply took a vacation. He went back to visit Bethany, back to the beach to catch a few more waves, and in a month's time he was back at Katahdin.

On his fourth attempt he made it through Maine, then New Hampshire, then Vermont, and when he reached Massachusetts, Andrew knew he would make it to Georgia. He had already survived the three states that had stymied him in the past; now all he had to do was keep his head down and put one foot in front of the other until he reached Springer Mountain.

In northern Pennsylvania, Andrew was doing just that, his gaze carefully focused on his foot placement amid the pointed rocks. The path resembled the mouth of a shark opening to engulf his surfboard, row upon row of sharp teeth waiting to consume him. As he carefully navigated the series of flesh-tearing protrusions, a low-hanging branch jabbed into his right eye. His face was scraped, his vision was blurry, and an aching pulse radiated from his forehead like a subwoofer.

By the time he reached the next road crossing, he had lost most of the vision in his right eye. He was convinced that he would have limited sight for the rest of his hike—if not the rest of his life—but he was determined not to quit or even take time off trail to see a doctor. He wrapped his swollen socket with a bandanna and kept hiking.

"I decided that I could finish the trail with one eye if I needed to," he said. After a day of gluey mucus streaming from the corner of his eye, followed by a day of crusty orange eyeliner surrounding his red pupil, Andrew's regained his sight and continued down the trail with two good eyes.

A few days later, near the town of Duncannon, Andrew's eye was better but the ball of his left foot felt as if it had a penknife lodged inside it.

"I knew something was seriously wrong with it," Andrew said. "I thought it was broken. I was convinced I had a stress fracture. Walking into town, I couldn't put any pressure on it. I knew this time I would have to go see a doctor and get it X-rayed. I thought my hike was over."

When he arrived on the outskirts of Duncannon and found J.B., he collapsed beside his friend in a fit of agony and despair. But J.B. wasn't the only one at the road crossing. Andrew had set a rule on his second attempt that no wives, girlfriends, or otherwise were allowed to join the crew. He was still hesitant about having females on his third endeavor, but his restrictions were less staunch this time. And when they passed within driving distance of the university where J.B.'s girlfriend attended med school, she was permitted to come out and see her man.

"It was a conjugal visit, which kind of pissed me off," Andrew said, "because I wasn't getting any. So I made a rule that she could come, but she had to wear a bikini. I didn't want J.B. to be the only one to benefit from it."

When Andrew came limping into town with a scowl on his face, there was a woman standing beside the support vehicle in her bathing suit. When she saw the pain that Andrew was experiencing, she dug through her luggage and brought out a long IV needle. She jammed it between Andrew's metatarsals and a small drop of fluid escaped. It was nothing more than a deeply embedded blister that didn't present itself. All the pain and anguish, the stress and pressure built up on the inside, were relieved by a simple release of fluid at the hands of a woman wearing a bikini.

"After that," he said, "I was a new man."

Andrew could not have set the record without J.B.—or J.B.'s girlfriend. At one point, even J.B.'s *father* came out to offer assistance.

When he reached the Southeast, Andrew was logging consistent fifty-mile days, but it was J.B. who was suffering from excruciating pain. For several weeks J.B. had been experiencing some discomfort behind one of his back molars. But recently, the discomfort had transitioned to a distracting ache and now, on record pace with just a few weeks left until the finish, J.B. felt as if the side of his face was going to fall off.

"J.B. was up all night gargling whiskey and taking painkillers so he could crew me the next day," said Andrew. "Finally we got to Virginia and J.B. begged his dad to take over crew duties for a day so that he could leave to find a dentist."

His dad obliged. J.B. made a beeline to the nearest dentist and had the tooth yanked for a hundred bucks. He was back on the trail crewing that evening.

"The catch is," Andrew said, "Jonboy could have kept the tooth if he had spent more time off trail. He gave up part of his body for me."

Andrew had invested a sizable amount going after his fourth record attempt. But so had his friend, and J.B. was going to do everything possible to make sure that Andrew made it to the finish this time.

When the support vehicle got a flat tire on the rural dirt roads of western North Carolina, J.B. quickly replaced it with the spare and kept driving. But then another tire blew, and he didn't have a way to fix it.

Andrew was depending on him, so J.B. kept driving, figuring he could make it up the mountain with one flat.

But then a third tire went . . . then another . . . and another. Incredibly, the truck blew five tires—all four wheels plus the spare. The severity of losing every tire calls to mind sabotage—or the back roads of western North Carolina. Or both.

If you piss off someone near where I live and he knows you're headed up a dirt road, there are likely to be nails in the gravel—sticking up. I'd guess that J.B. and Andrew were collateral damage to some good old-fashioned redneck revenge. (Welcome to the South, y'all.)

When Andrew arrived at the trailhead, he saw the truck resting on its rims, but J.B. assured his friend that he would take care of everything.

That night, Andrew and J.B. sat quietly next to each other on camping pads that were stretched out in the truck bed of the lame pickup. For dinner, they spooned cold Chef Boyardee out of cans by headlamp, and then they lay down, pulled their sleeping bags up to their chins, and bivvied out underneath the stars. They woke before the sun came out, as they always did, and then both set out in the dark on what Andrew calls "the most critical day of the record."

Andrew hiked sixteen miles, and J.B. drove four times as far on flats. Three and a half hours later, J.B. and the Tacoma were waiting at the entrance to the Smoky Mountain National Park with four freshly patched and inflated tires.

Andrew's tone changed as he recounted the story, momentarily trading bravado for a hint of sentimentality. "Jonboy was going to do whatever it took to get us there."

Five days after fixing the tires, the two friends found themselves in an unfamiliar position. The end.

"I knew what I wanted at the end of that hike. I knew who I wanted to be there. I just wanted it to be me and Jonboy," he said. "That's it."

Under a coal-black sky on August 1, 2005, Andrew and J.B. climbed Springer Mountain together. They finished in Georgia and claimed the overall record on the AT, surpassing Pete Palmer's mark by more than twenty-four hours.

When they walked off Springer Mountain and into the forest service parking lot, J.B. pulled a six-pack of beer from the ice cooler. He had occupied his time between road crossings that day with one final Herculean task, trying to find beer in a dry county.

While J.B. searched for his can opener, Andrew went to the edge of the forest and bent down to gather fallen branches and collect dry twigs off the ground. As he squatted, his thighs screamed with lactic acid. He was exhausted. The bundle of kindling he toted to the fire pit felt like a fallen tree in his arms. But this was a blissful fatigue. He had accomplished his goal. Starting the fire would be the last physical task required before reclining in the dark with his best friend and drinking in their accomplishment.

Andrew placed the smallest twigs in a pyramid formation and stuck a few dry leaves between the sticks. He struck a match and held it at the base of his creation. An orange line started eating away at the brown leaves. Andrew added the larger branches over the kindling. Then he put his hands on the earth and lowered his head to meet them. He gently blew life into the decaying matter and watched as the orange sparks spread their light and heat. Then, using his lungs as bellows, he swallowed the night sky in preparation for a large exhalation, but in the process of taking in oxygen he also inhaled some of the smoke.

"I don't know what was in it," he said, "but all of sudden I got a lungful and I thought I was going to die. I curled up in a fetal position and told J.B. to turn off the music and get rid of the beer. It felt like I was having a heart attack. I was shivering with cold sweats and chills. I'd hiked close to fifty miles a day all summer and that was the worst I'd felt the entire trip. Jonboy sat right beside me in the camp chair. When I finally stopped convulsing, he helped me into the tent around 4:00 a.m."

I laughed.

"What's so funny?" Andrew asked indignantly.

"Well," I said, "you probably gathered some laurel or rhododendron branches and inhaled toxic smoke."

"And that's funny to you?"

"Well, it's just ironic that of all the smoke you've inhaled in your life it was the campfire at the base of Springer Mountain that nearly killed you."

Andrew grinned, nodded, and said, "Yeah, I see your point."

After thirty years of being told that he was not good enough, Andrew Thompson finally found his liberation by running into the woods, breaking the barriers of endurance, and proving to everyone—and most important, to himself—that he *was* good enough.

On the surface, the record had demanded a molar, a med student in a bikini, the better part of three summers, and past reckonings with winter storms and life-sucking mud. But Andrew's record was also rooted in twenty-one years of Christian matriculation, church on Sundays (and Wednesdays), a strict father, an oft-complacent mother, and a failed marriage—and the ability to let that all go in order to arrive at Springer Mountain.

The thing about a long, grueling journey is that it strips away who you're not and allows you to discover what's left—or who's left. One damn good reason to pursue endurance—and choose suffering—is to get to know yourself inside and out. When you reach that moment where you gave more than you thought you had and accomplished more than you thought you could, it's clear who you are.

The first time I met Andrew Thompson was when we crossed paths on the Appalachian Trail. The next encounter was two and a half years later at David Horton's Mountain Masochist. Andrew and J.B. were running the race together.

They did not, however, begin the race with the 298 other registered participants.

Instead, Andrew and J.B. started twelve hours before everyone else—at the finish line. Then they ran fifty miles, mostly in the dark, to reach the starting line. Once they reached the race's official origin, they toed the line with the rest of the ultrarunners. When the gunshot rang out into the night sky, they turned around and ran fifty miles back the way they had come the night before.

It was my first fifty-mile race and I was ecstatic to finish. Yet I felt my result—everyone's result—was diminished ever so slightly by the fact that J.B. and Andrew had finished the course twice. If Andrew wanted to make his fastest known time on the AT seem more intimidating and impressive than it already was, he did it by finishing a *double* Mountain Masochist in less than twenty-four hours.

But as I learned at my first ultramarathon, when I sat at a picnic table drinking prerace beers with the elite runners, being a participant at these races means that you often have the opportunity to rub shoulders with greatness. Now here I was at the Mountain Masochist standing in the shadows of people such as David Horton, Andrew Thompson, and J.B. They were my idols of long-distance adventures. And I knew my place in their midst; I was a fan, certainly not their competition.

I didn't think I could go neck and neck with Andrew Thompson, so I decided to try to stalk him. Even if his record was out of reach, I could still follow in his footprints.

In 2008, I went back to the Appalachian Trail for the second time. With all these different trail attempts, thru hikes, and races it can get confusing, so let me clarify. I have hiked the entire AT three times: The first was a traditional thru hike. My last hike set the overall FKT for men and women. And the one in between the two was . . . well, it was in between the two. You could say I was dipping my toes into trail records.

At that time the fastest known time for a female stood at

ninety-nine days and was a mark established by an unsupported ul-tralight backpacker who had completed a traditional thru hike with her husband. If I finished anywhere south of that, I could establish a new female record. The goal seemed achievable.

I will never forget coming out at a road crossing in the latter stages of my hike. Brew was grinning from ear to ear as he handed me his cell phone and told me to listen to the message.

"Hey, Brew, this is Andrew Thompson calling from Hanover, New Hampshire. I met Jen a couple times over the years at Horton's races and I hold the speed record on the Appalachian Trail. I was just calling to tell her that she needs to fucking get after it. She's got my full support. She is putting on a hell of a clinic out there on the trail. I know how tough it is so tell her to kick some ass . . . and I've got her back . . . and I'm *so* proud of her. I'm so proud of you guys. So give me a call back and tell me what's going on. See ya."

With a little prodding from David Horton, Andrew had called to commend my efforts. And I know verbatim what the message says because eight years later Brew still has the recording.

I finished the trail in fifty-seven days and set the women's FKT. Still, I was a full ten days behind Andrew's time. To put that into perspective, if we had started our hikes at the same time, I would still have had 380 miles to go when he reached the finish. When a runner gets passed on a track, he is lapped. Andrew Thompson's record was more than a proverbial lap ahead of my time. It was a full state. I got stated.

That same summer a celebrated ultrarunner named Karl Meltzer, the man who had won more one-hundred-mile races than anyone else in history, tried to surpass Andrew's mark. He had ample re-sources and a sponsorship the likes of which the Appalachian Trail had never seen. Still, he finished in fifty-four days, a full week behind the current record. Andrew was no longer on the AT, he was sitting at home drinking beer, but he continued to outpace everyone.

The next spring, Andrew took another step in imitating David

Horton and intimidating his ultrarunning competitors when he finished the hundred-mile Barkley Marathon. In the world of FKTs, Barkley appears more than any other race. It is arguably the most difficult hundred-mile race and it is universally regarded as the one with the most character.

The application fee for Barkley is $1.60 plus a handwritten essay on why you should be allowed to run the race. If you are chosen as a participant, the cost of entry is a license plate from your home state. The race starts when the director blows into a large conch shell—and he can decide to do that whenever he wants. Along the route you are forced to search for books that the race director has hidden in the forest and tear out specified pages. When your race ends, and it will almost certainly end before the finish line, you receive a bugle serenade of Taps—the tune of choice at flag lowerings, military funerals, and Barkley. The fact that so many long-distance record holders have been successful finishing the eccentric sixty-hour race when so few others have suggests that there is a strong connection between suffering at Barkley and surviving an FKT.

The fact that the race has a two-and-a-half-day cutoff means that participants can average less than two miles per hour and still finish. Yet in most years, no one will complete the race. That is because it is less of a run and more of a scramble up and down the limestone cliffs of central Tennessee and because the race director takes great pride in turning his event into a psychological labyrinth. Of the fourteen men who have exited the unmarked maze of rock outcroppings, deciduous trees, and briars, six of them are known for their FKT resumes, including David Horton, Andrew Thompson, and his closest friend, J.B.

Besides providing incredible support to Andrew, J.B. is an accomplished endurance athlete in his own right. He finished Barkley and also set the record on Vermont's 272-mile Long Trail. Andrew crewed for him on both endeavors.

The parallels between Barkley and FKTs should in no way lead people, particularly my husband and mother, to believe that I have illusions about competing at Barkley. What it means is that there is an elite fraternity forming of long-trail record holders and Barkley finishers. They are the untouchables. They walk around ultra events with chips on their shoulders, but not because they are going to win the race. These guys aren't known for being the fastest. They are known for being the toughest. They win at intimidation.

That's why I felt nervous, scared, and like a complete fool when I emailed Andrew to let him know that I was going after his record.

"I didn't think you had a chance in hell," he told me while lounging in the comfort of his living room, a double IPA in hand.

I'd reached out to Andrew before trying for his record because I wanted to adhere to FKT etiquette and because I respected him and wanted to be transparent. Andrew immediately wrote back to wish me luck, adding that if I needed the numbers or daily mileages from his 2005 hike, he would be happy to share them. He also mentioned that if he was in town, he would come hike with me when I passed through New Hampshire.

"You were so nice about it," I said.

"I was just doing the math," he replied. "There's a huge gap between forty-seven days and fifty-seven days. I mean, several *hundred* miles."

"I know," I said a bit smugly.

Andrew laughed. "I told you about the day I knew you were going to set the record, right?"

I nodded, but he commenced with the story anyway.

"I knew once you got down South that the record was yours. I took a hike on the AT up to Mount Cube. By the time I came off that mountain I'd said good-bye to the record. I held it for six years—to the day. It was time to move on.

"That night when Bethany came home, she was wearing her sunglasses and looked really pretty . . ."

Andrew was gazing out the window as if he could envision his wife driving home from work at that very moment.

"Hold on a second," he said.

Then he stood up and left the living room. I thought he was going to find a photo album or some sentimental memento to complement his story, but I nearly hit the roof when I heard a .22-caliber rifle ring out in the front yard.

Andrew stomped back into the house, took off his garden shoes, and turned to the border collie.

"Go get it, Bobby."

The dog ran out the door as Andrew came in and plopped back down on the sofa. Taking a swig from his beer, he matter-of-factly said, "Red squirrel; dead squirrel. Now where was I?"

I looked out the window to see his dog chomping on a limp carcass beneath a swaying bird feeder.

"Um . . . the record . . . Bethany . . . she was about to tell you . . ."

"Oh yeah, that's right. She was about to tell me she was pregnant. She walked up the driveway with a big smile on her face and when she took off her shades I knew there was something going on.

"I looked at her and said, 'Oh, my God, you're pregnant.' She nodded. That's the moment I found out I was going to be a father."

The fall after Brew and I surpassed the mark of Andrew and J.B., we ran into them, once again, at the Mountain Masochist. When Andrew saw me, he immediately left his group of friends, walked straight toward me, and then engulfed me in his arms.

"Do you remember that?" I asked. "You congratulated me on the record and then you gave me a present. It was a wrapped picture frame that had a photo we had taken together at Masochist the year before. I thought it was so classy of you. Then you said, 'The AT is an adventure, but just remember your greatest adventures are still ahead.' You were referring to your son and I thought it was so sweet. It made me want to start my family pronto. Less than a year later, Brew and I welcomed Charley (our daughter) into the world."

Andrew's face lit up with joy and he let out a sadistic howl.

"Payback's a bitch, isn't it? That's the same shit I told Jonboy. I didn't want to be the only one taking care of a kid. And now I've got two of them. It's miserable! That's why I talk all my friends into having another one.

"You should have seen all the pictures I texted to J.B.'s woman of my two boys playing, telling her she and J.B. needed to have another one, saying how sweet it is when they play together. Now J.B.'s stuck taking care of a second and texting me pictures of an empty whiskey glass. By the way, he's texting me those pictures midmorning. *Midmorning.*"

On cue, Andrew's youngest came marching down the steps post-nap calling for his daddy.

"Come're, baby," Andrew said as he reached out his arms.

The hefty toddler climbed up in his dad's lap and threw his rounded arms around Andrew's neck. Andrew put his beer down and gently stroked his son's back.

"Don't you think it's a little like the trail?" I asked. "Don't you think that amid the daily grind there are sunsets, and views, and moments like this—when a snuggle makes you realize that you are the center of this kid's whole world—that make the misery worthwhile."

Andrew turned to kiss his son's cheek, then looked back at me

"Maybe," he said with a smile.

There is a special relationship between a record setter and the person who breaks his or her record. In one sense, you are great adversaries, but in another you share the closest of bonds with them. Andrew Thompson pushed me to be my best physical self on the trail. Just as important, and somewhat surprisingly, he also taught me how to be gracious off of it. Whereas Warren and Horton were the ones who taught me how to set a record, it was Andrew who showed me how to let go.

In 2011, I set the FKT for men and women and I cut twenty-six hours off the mark that Andrew and J.B. had set. The one thing I dreaded after reaching Springer Mountain was talking to Andrew. I

knew that he would call or email. It wasn't required; it wasn't a part
of the understood FKT rules. But I knew it was coming. It felt awkward for someone whom I had looked up to for so long to congratulate me on breaking his record. I didn't want him to feel compelled to
say nice things that he didn't mean.

So when I saw an email from him pop up in my inbox, I cringed.
The subject line had a smiley face and I dreaded opening the message
to work my way painfully through his obligatory concession.

But when I finally worked up the courage to click on it, I called for
Brew and started laughing out loud. The entire message contained
two words:

"You Bitch!" Followed by another smiling emoji.

It was impressive that Andrew could say so much—and be completely honest—with a pair of words. He'd managed to acknowledge
my accomplishment, admit his attachment to the record, and prevent
any future awkwardness, all the while complimenting me with an
insult.

The kinship I feel for Andrew is disproportionate to the limited
time we have spent together. In a typical year, I *may* see Andrew
once, and if I do see him, it is in Lynchburg at David Horton's fall
classic. He is always warm and welcoming, but we never visit long
because he is there to be with his best friends. It is the one weekend
each year when Andrew, J.B., and their close-knit group of friends
travel from across the country to run fifty miles together and recap
the experiences of the past year, one step at a time. It is a tradition
that dates back twenty years.

Andrew is a great long-distance friend, partly because of his prolific texting habits. Each summer, when someone sets out for an AT
FKT attempt, I know that I will start getting text updates from Andrew. And with each new contender he is unabashed with his criticism and his humor. In a sport without trophies, one of the best
rewards is sitting back and watching other people suffer as they try to
surpass your mark.

In 2015, it felt appropriate to learn that my record had fallen via a text from Andrew. I had taken his record, and now he was letting me know that someone else had surpassed mine.

"Jurek just summited Katahdin," he wrote. "He beat you by three hours. Sorry."

And then a few seconds later a follow-up message: "I hope you know your pace almost fucking killed him."

Andrew always finds a way to make you smile.

It's ironic that despite his painful upbringing in the church, the one thing I admire most about Andrew Thompson is typically seen as a Christian ideal: Even more than his athletic prowess and his charismatic personality, Andrew demonstrates an uncanny ability to forgive.

He was completely forthcoming about the negative aspects of his upbringing and his parents' religion, and in the next breath he volunteered how grateful he was for the relationship he shared with his mother and father as an adult.

During my stay at his house, he was actively packing for a weekend with his mom and siblings at a nearby lake. Both his mother and his in-laws live nearby, allowing them to have a close relationship with their grandsons—and with Andrew and Bethany. But his father switched from preaching to hospice care a long time ago and now lives in Florida with his girlfriend.

"The last time I was down there with the boys," Andrew said, "I asked my dad, 'Don't you think that was kind of a bizarre twelve years?' Talking about my childhood. I mean, he was so intense. He was like me, animated and intense. Now, he's lost all that. He's super kind and laid back."

A smirk came over Andrew's face. "I've never been handed as many joints as when I was at my dad's house. And I had the boys with me. But, I'm telling you, he is the best hospice end-of-life care giver ever. He used to tell people that he had all the answers; now he just listens."

For Andrew, the long path to happiness has included a difficult upbringing, a divorce, and three failed record attempts. But ultimately, Andrew says, "It's all good." He shows us the best way to move forward is not to forsake the past, but to forgive it—and yourself.

"Looking back on life, looking back on the trail, hell . . . seeing a white blaze, it's like seeing an old friend, an *old* friend," he says. "It's kinda like looking at a picture of an ex-girlfriend. You think about why it went wrong back then, all the fights and the stupid stuff. Then you really look at this girl and think, 'I loved this girl . . . and I still love this girl.'

"People get so freakin' defeated and deflated by stuff," he said. "I understand that mental illness is a real thing. I don't need to go too far down that road. But like, okay, here's a bad life . . . your toddler being killed in Syria. Okay? *That's* called a bad life, all right?

"We've got it made. But stuff still happens; this is life. Things are gonna go bad. You're gonna pop a tire on your car, you're gonna turn the key one morning and the car's not going to start. That's everyday stuff. You deal with it. Drink some water. Go for a run. Have an attitude adjustment and stop thinking so goddamn much.

"I like to think of it as just happily rolling with the punches that life throws at you. If you are a life lover, you love it all, you take it all. You hike through that five-hour rainstorm when your hands are so freakin' numb that you can't operate your zipper because you know when that sucker's over, the sun's gonna come out and when it does you're gonna be sucking up all that warmth. And you're gonna be like, 'While that rainstorm was raging hell for five hours, I just hiked twenty miles. And now, I've come out the other end and I'm good to go.'"

As with Scott Williamson, the trail taught Andrew more than he ever learned in school. "The trail is a big-boy education," he said. "Think of it. You can't recite to me your class schedule senior year in college; you probably don't even know what classes you *took*. But you can sit here and give me a litany of lessons you learned on the trail . . . that affect you *every day* and affect your actions and choices and how you raise your kids, and the direction you take in life. You know? Some of that has to do with speed . . . but most of it doesn't."

And whereas religious failed him, it was running and hiking long distances that showed Andrew how to trust others (or at a minimum J.B.), believe in himself, and uncover a love for the daily grind.

CHAPTER SEVEN

Wife, Mother, Record Setter

"We are never doing that again!"
—My husband, Brew Davis

O n July 31, 2011, I walked off Springer Mountain hand in hand with Brew. We had just surpassed Andrew Thompson's record on the Appalachian Trail. The new mark stood at 46 days, 11 hours, and 20 minutes—an average of 47 miles per day. It was the first time that a female had claimed the overall title on the AT—and the first time a woman had reigned on one of the long long-distance trails in the United States. There had been a supreme title held by Sue Johnston on the shorter, 211-mile John Muir Trail in 2007. But beyond that feat, I am unaware of another woman holding an FKT on a National Scenic Trail before 2011.

The most common question I received after I set the record was *not* how we accomplished the feat, what we learned during the endeavor, or what it meant to us as a couple. Instead, everyone wanted to know "What's next?"

I have not tried for any other fastest known time and I have not participated in any ultramarathons or organized races since.

After 2011, I turned my attention to work and family. Because I have a liking for green spaces, I have a large yard that requires more mowing than I would like. I also own and manage a hiking company with employees and guides, and that requires constant supervision, not to mention an unsettling amount of liability. Most days, I look longingly out the window at a lawn that needs to be mowed and I wonder how a career built on getting people outdoors can demand so much time behind a computer and on the phone.

In 2013, I welcomed my daughter into the world, and in the process of working on this book, we added a little boy. Parenting feels like a backpacking trip that never ends; it is both rewarding and brutal. Then there is marriage. Although my husband is nearly perfect (ahem, in the eyes of his mother), we still struggle daily to find copacetic methods of working together, coparenting, managing household chores, and maintaining our relationship.

In many ways, I feel as if I have been hard at work. Yet when I visit trail folks like Andrew and Scott, I feel as if I have been completely dormant. My FKT contemporaries are in much better shape than I am, they are actively planning and executing adventures, they seemingly have a better work-life balance, and most important, they have kept a part of themselves that I have let go: Physical challenges and extended time outdoors are still very much an integral part of their lives. Even David Horton, who is in his midsixties, is more active than I am.

At the moment, in terms of my athletic output, I feel more like Warren Doyle than any other record setter I know. Credit where credit is due, Warren still hikes and goes to contra dances several nights a week. Nonetheless, it is depressing to feel that you are on a par with a man in his sixties who refers to McDonald's as his "home office."

Delving into the personalities and stories of fastest known times has been a more difficult and introspective journey than I anticipated. For the most part I have felt out of place. And yet, I still find my name on the same list as everyone else's. After Warren, David, and Andrew, right alongside the unsupported feats of Scott and others, I am—or at least I was—a record holder.

More and more I ask myself, "How did I claim that spot and why do I feel so far removed from everyone else?"

As with Warren and Scott, I discovered thru hiking at a formative age, and it forever changed my life.

After graduating from college in Alabama I was offered a job as a programming organizer for children with special needs. It was a position I would have gladly accepted—in another six months. But without taking a moment to consider the proposition, I turned it down. The director of the organization, and the supervisor at my part-time job, was taken aback, if not altogether offended.

"Why?" he asked.

"Because I'm planning to hike the Appalachian Trail," I responded.

"Well," he replied, "I hope you take some time and really think about what it is that you're running away from."

I nodded and walked out of his office. I wasn't yet used to defending my hike and I didn't know what to say. Now, I am very comfortable looking folks in the eyes and saying, "Hiking is not escapism; it's realism. The people who choose to spend time outdoors are not running away from anything; we are returning to where we belong."

I couldn't accept a job right out of college because—to repeat what I have heard from nearly every thru hiker I know—I wasn't yet done with my education.

My first thru hike on the Appalachian Trail took nearly half a year to complete. It was difficult from day one and varied from that point forward in its degree of difficulty; it was never easy.

One of my immediate observations was that you don't realize how often it rains until you live outside. A week and a half into the hike, I had already been wet more days than not. That afternoon I sought cover under the roof of a trail shelter during a thunderstorm. Damp and chilled from walking all day in bad weather, I went behind the building where I could change into my dry long johns in privacy—and away from ten or so male hikers huddled inside the structure.

I was hugging up against the wooden beams of the building, trying to remain under the protection of the overhanging metal roof. Just as I lifted my hands over my head to strip off a pullover fleece, there was a flash of light and suddenly it felt as if I were being lashed by an electric fence. A hot dagger traveled from my raised arms, down my spine, into my legs, and out of my body. The shelter had taken a direct hit from the lightning, and a portion of the current jumped into the tall, thin, conductor who was reaching her hands toward the sky.

The pain was gone in seconds, but the emotional shock remained. For a moment, I stood there in disbelief. Then I looked down at my legs and stretched out my arms to make sure I was okay. I continued a short self-assessment, but when I didn't see any negative side effects, I took a few deep breaths and then kept getting dressed. I was fortunate; the only lasting impact of the lightning strike was that I developed a serious respect for electrical storms.

The National Weather Service reports that the odds of getting struck by lightning are 1 in 13,500. I'm sure it's higher than that for hikers. Off the top of my head I can rattle off five friends who have stories of being, at a minimum, buzzed. If you do get hit, your chances of surviving are high, around 90 percent, but I'm still not willing to roll the dice. So now I'm trained in CPR and I've taught dozens of folks the proper position and safest locations to take when lightning is near.

In Great Smoky Mountains National Park, I backpacked eighteen miles through a blizzard. The snow and sleet were biting. As I hiked across an exposed ridgeline I lowered my head, closed my left eye, and tucked my chin down and away from the sinister wind. When I reentered the protection of the forest, I lifted my head but I couldn't open my eye. It had frozen shut. Trying to find the trail's iconic white blazes in a blizzard was nearly impossible with perfect vision, let alone limited eyesight.

I took off the wool socks I used as mittens, pawed at my eyelids, and picked the ice off my face so I could see clearly again. Then I once again peered at the white trees, white boulders, and white ground, trying to decipher the trail. I turned my head to look at the footsteps behind me and then directed my attention to the unbroken snow before me. I took in a heavy cold breath and kept walking.

One of the most important lessons the trail taught me is that I need vision and want direction. It doesn't matter how hard you are working if you are walking the wrong way.

The most challenging ailments were not experienced in seconds or even hours, but in days and weeks. The trail dished out long term-discomfort: blisters that wouldn't heal, shoulders that ached under the constant weight of my pack, muscle and joint pains that were aggravated by . . . wait for it . . . hiking, trench foot caused by too much rain, and an uncomfortable numbness shooting down my right leg whose cause I never pinpointed. There are pains that you can work through fairly quickly, but most of the complaints you carry with you as part and parcel of the journey.

The trail presented an abundance of social challenges and awkward situations, as well. Things like sleeping next to strangers in a shelter, sleeping next to strangers in a shelter who snore and pass gas all night, or sleeping in a shelter by myself and wondering if a stranger would arrive in the middle of the night.

When I started the journey, I was worried that I would be lonely for much of my time on the trail. What I found is that loneliness often hits harder in a crowd—at school or in the workplace, a packed bar or a party—than alone in the woods. I came to believe that solitude was something to be sought, not avoided. I learned to embrace the time to myself and occasionally found it difficult to maintain.

In Virginia I gained an unwelcome hiking companion. I met a nice enough young man around my age, and after exchanging the usual hiker pleasantries he followed on my heels for six days. Six days! The attention he bestowed quickly shifted from flattering to stifling. I tried everything I could think of to create space, but after I failed to shake him with obvious hints and erratic pacing tactics, I ultimately tried to escape from him by hiding beneath a rhododendron bush. In retrospect, I wish that I had turned to him and plainly stated, "I don't want to hike with you anymore." A more direct approach would probably have proven effective. It certainly would have been more dignified than lying facedown in the dirt underneath a mountain shrub! But because of my cowardice and a dense rhododendron thicket, I'll never know.

The hardest day of my hike and one of the most difficult days of my life occurred in New Jersey, when I came across the body of a man who had committed suicide. I was hiking by myself and came across a dead body, bound in rope and hanging from the rafters of a picnic pavilion. I felt my stomach drop out of my body. I was terrified, traumatized. I turned and ran. At some point, I stopped and called the cops. The police met me on the trail and then asked me questions for ten to fifteen minutes. After scribbling down my answers on a notepad, an officer turned and said, "So is this your first stiff?"

I looked at him in horror.

A fellow officer noticed my aghast look and gave his coworker an admonishing nudge. Then he said, "Sorry about that, miss. At this point, I think we have what we need. You can keep hiking now."

Keep hiking? . . . Now?

I felt like a ball of rubber bands knotted up with frustration, anger, and confusion. I didn't know if I could keep hiking, or if I *wanted* to keep hiking. But without knowing what else to do, I stood up and put one foot in front of the other.

Over a decade later, I can still recall every minute detail of a scene that I took in for just a split second. I remember the color of the young man's clothes, the angle of his feet pointing toward the floor, and the sound of the rope swaying gently back and forth. I remember nuances of setting to the point that even today scent and sound are palpable.

When people talk casually about suicide, I tear up. When I watch a movie scene portraying or even discussing suicide, I have to close my eyes and ears. More than a decade later, I'll still round a turn on the Appalachian Trail and experience a visceral flashback. I will forever be affected by the suicide of a person I didn't even know.

But through that experience, I learned that physical motion is a form of therapy. There is power to be found in taking a next step. The fact that my body could keep hiking down the trail gave me hope that my thoughts and emotions would be able to move forward as well.

For seventeen hundred miles I thought surely, at some point, the trail would get easier. Then I got to Vermont and I discovered, in the words of Andrew Thompson, life-sucking mud. I cried unabashedly as I walked through shoe-slurping muck, choking humidity, and clouds of biting blackflies hovering overhead. I had persevered through a lightning strike, snow, a stalker, and a suicide. I had passed through twelve states, with the two hardest still to come. The conditions were ever changing but never what I wanted.

I finally accepted that the Appalachian Trail was not going to change to meet my needs; I couldn't control the trail. So after twenty weeks of hiking, at last I started to adapt to my environment.

Novice thru hikers usually discard unnecessary gear within several dozen miles of Springer Mountain in Georgia. It took months for me to discard my sense of self-importance and learn that I couldn't hike with the weight of my pride. Instead of merely reacting to the trail and to others, I finally embraced how to cry and laugh for myself—and by myself. I also realized I couldn't keep going without asking for help. I couldn't ask for help if I didn't trust people, and I couldn't trust people unless I let go of my preconceived notions and stereotypes.

When I finished my hike, I was a different person—a better person. But I also never wanted to hike another long-distance trail in my life. Instead of feeling hooked, I felt shattered and exhausted. I could hardly wait to start an office job—with air-conditioning, indoor plumbing, and a communal coffee pot.

I applied for work at a history museum and was offered the job. I was surrounded by fascinating guests and coworkers; it was everything that I thought I wanted in a work position. I was following the trajectory my life was heading before the last 2,189 miles. I should have been happy, I should have been content, but weeks passed, then months, and all I could think about was the trail.

Warren had warned me, "The AT will change you." He was right.

When I was sitting at my desk, I missed being in nature. When I was lying in bed at night and staring at the ceiling, I missed being serenaded by insects and falling asleep as soon as I closed my eyelids. And even though I was taking showers, combing my hair, putting on makeup, and wearing clean clothes—not to mention deodorant—I missed how beautiful I felt when I was hiking.

When I was hiking I rarely saw my reflection and I didn't have advertisements, media, or social networks telling me what I should look like. Consequently, I started to see myself, literally and figuratively, in a new light, that is, through the interactions I had with other hikers. If I was kind, or funny, if I made someone else smile, that was my reflection; that made me feel beautiful. Growing up, I had always thought that nature was beautiful, but I had never seen myself as a part of nature. I had never seen myself as a part of all that beauty— until I hiked the trail.

After hiking through fourteen states and after covering more than two thousand miles, I no longer based my self-worth on how I looked. Instead I started to gain confidence as a result of what I could do. The trail made me realize I could do much more than I once thought possible. And I wanted to do more, I wanted to feel *that* beautiful again. I wanted to keep hiking.

When I first started backpacking, I didn't think of the trail as a competitive environment. In fact, I still don't. In the beginning, my greatest adversary was my own sense of self, and it still is. Self-consciousness and self-imposed limitations are what I spend most of my time trying to outrun. But with each new hike I undertake, I also find myself toward the front of the thru-hiking pack and surrounded by men.

I have always loved trying to keep up with the boys. When I was little I thought I was one of them. In my family, I was the youngest of three children and the only girl. I grew up dressing in my brothers' hand-me-downs. I had a closely trimmed (read "boys'") haircut that my mom claims was stylish in the mid-eighties. And when I underwent potty training, my parents told me I tried to stand up and use the toilet just like my brothers. (After being told for most of my life that women should sit or squat to pee, I can now do it standing up with my backpack on as well, so I guess my childhood efforts have come in handy.)

My early years were spent with my parents and two older brothers in a rustic home that sat high on a mountainside in rural western North Carolina. We had a garden in the backyard that was bordered by blackberry and raspberry bushes. While picking that sweet fruit as a child, I remember discovering the coarse black fur of some ursine forager tangled on a nearby fence.

My brothers and I shared a seemingly gargantuan sandbox in the front yard of our house. After a summer rainstorm, we would build bunkers, then fashion sand balls, which also happened to be filled with sticks and rocks. When everyone's redoubt was well stocked, we commenced with a sand ball fight of epic proportions, battles that always resulted in injuries and tears. I was almost always the one crying.

One of the earliest memories I have of my mother is taking evening walks with her down the long, unpaved driveway that led to the road. I recall on more than one occasion spotting a tan and brown copperhead soaking up the waning warmth of the gravel on the roadway. My mother and I would then race back to the house, hop into the jeep, and drive down the road, trying to flatten it. It wasn't that my mother hated snakes, but she was concerned about protecting her children and the resident summer campers.

My childhood home was on the same property as the camp my father owned and operated. It was a boys' camp. Each summer I was surrounded by hundreds of male campers and counselors who traveled from across the country and the world to go on backpacking trips, swim in mountain lakes, and ride horses.

I was younger than the youngest campers by several years, but I was determined not to be left out. I went to all the activities with the boys. I remember crying at riflery because I hated the crack of the guns, but at the same time I refused to leave. I never hit the target at archery and left with huge red welts on the inside of my left arm. At the nature hut, I let the ring-neck snakes weave around my fingers and when I held the pet rat I remember it twirled its tail like a helicopter blade. There is no better place for a child to grow up than at a summer camp.

Then when I was in first grade, my father sold the camp and we moved into town. My childhood from that point forward was filled with the traditional sports, after-school clubs, homework, and sleepovers at friends' houses. I still spent my summers at camp, but this was an all-girls sleepaway camp where the activities included glass bead making and modeling (think high fashion, not toy airplanes). I loved my weeks at sleepaway camp, but it wasn't the wilderness environment where I had spent my early years. We had left behind our home on the mountain, but a part of me always wanted to go back.

When I was twenty-one years old, my father, beaming with pride, dropped me off in the middle of a national forest in Georgia. When I got out of his truck, he promised to pick me up again, but only if I made it all the way to Maine. My mother worried constantly about me when I started hiking; she still does. But it was the first home they provided for me, where it was okay to splash in puddles and throw sand balls, where I could hold rats and ring-neck snakes, where I could find bear fur in the berry patch and snakes sunning themselves on the gravel driveway that made those first few steps feel like a homecoming.

The great thing about finding a home on the trail is that you can live anywhere. After my first thru hike, I backpacked the Pacific Crest Trail, Vermont's Long Trail, and a handful of international hikes. But, in 2008, I returned to the Appalachian Trail, this time with my husband. After I met Brew, getting married was not a difficult decision. I knew after a few dates that I wanted to spend the rest of my life with him. After just five months, we were engaged.

After we had been together for a total of ten months, we were married on a beautiful mountain in Virginia. Twelve days later we hiked Katahdin together and I commenced a southbound hike, hoping to establish a women's record.

Looking back, I wish I had better reasons for trying to set the record. But the hike was more or less a utilitarian effort. Brew was a schoolteacher who was not interested in long-distance backpacking, yet. He did love to go on day hikes, though, and road trips, especially if he could fit in visits to some Civil War battlefields and craft breweries. As we were newlyweds who had only courted for ten months, the thought of being separated for a season seemed unbearable. Besides, I told Brew on one of our very first dates that before settling down I wanted—I needed—to hike the Appalachian Trail just *one* more time.

On a supported hike, I could spend all day on the trail and Brew could alternate between hiking stretches with me and sightseeing. Without the weight of a full pack or task of resupplying, I could complete the trail faster and align the dates with Brew's summer vacation. And we could get it out of my system once and for all. The women's record just happened to be there. No one had tried for it before and I knew that as long as I didn't get injured, I would likely set the mark.

Fifty-seven days later we reached Springer Mountain. I had set the women's FKT. But when we walked off Springer Mountain, I realized that there was something more to a trail record than a title; there was also a record-setting experience, and I knew I had missed out on that.

I stayed well within my comfort zone for the duration of the hike, starting each morning when the sun came up and finishing by dusk. I never set a specific goal for the day, the week, or even the summer. I figured that if I maximized daylight and finished the trail in less than three months, it would be a smashing success.

When David Horton came out to help that summer he kept telling me that I was making it look too easy and that I was having too much fun. But at the same time something in his eyes suggested that I wasn't enjoying it *enough*. That I wasn't working hard enough to really, truly be getting the most out of the experience.

David and Warren were both there as I neared the finish. Their anticipation of the end surpassed my own. They were reliving something that I had not fully experienced.

"You could end this record with a real exclamation mark," said Horton.

Warren agreed, "Ending with a sixty-mile day would really make a statement. But that means you are going to have to night hike."

"But what if I trip and get injured or lost in the darkness?" I asked. I hadn't spent much time night hiking that summer and felt hesitant and less enthusiastic than my two compatriots.

"I know the way," said Warren. "You can point your headlamp at the back of my shoes and follow me."

Warren persuaded me to start at 2:00 a.m. and hike with him under the stars. For twelve miles, we walked together through the cool of the night and the gentle noises of all things nocturnal. It was one of the most memorable and rewarding experiences of the summer. When morning broke, I was left to wonder why I had never spent more time exploring the trail after dark. Thousands of miles into this relationship there was a whole different aspect of the wilderness that I had been unaware of until then.

At the final mountain, I remember how strong and happy I felt as I snapped photos and signed the last register. We dawdled on the summit, taking it in, then I bounded down the mountain to enjoy a restaurant meal with the family members and friends who had come to the finish. We drove back to Asheville that evening and after taking two days to rest and get organized, I went back to my regular work and exercise routine.

There was no doubt in my mind that I could have given more that summer. Almost immediately I knew that I should have completed the trail in a shorter time. So why hadn't I?

There were a lot of excuses—not the least of which was being on a quasi-honeymoon—but to be brutally honest, the primary reason I didn't try harder was that I was a woman. I subconsciously believed that records had to be split by gender. I decided before I ever started that I couldn't compete with the men, so I limited myself to establishing the female mark instead. If I had been a male I would have had an entirely different mind-set that summer.

My thought process was not entirely unscientific or without cultural bias. Professional athletics in the United States suggest that women's sport are separate—and not equal. Professional female athletes have had to fight for exposure, pay, and most of all respect.

I had been placed on athletic teams from elementary school clear through to my college years. Growing up in youth leagues, I knew that my male counterparts were typically faster and stronger than I was. Even if I trained harder and wanted it more, they could still outmuscle me. But after hiking the trail in fifty-seven days, I realized that completing a journey of 2,189 miles quickly had little to do with speed and strength. It was a lot more about strategy and teamwork, logistics and good luck, but most of all it was about endurance. I knew I couldn't outmuscle the men, but after that fifty-seven-day hike, I started to wonder if I could outlast them.

Much as with my first thru hike on the Appalachian Trail, when I walked off Springer Mountain I never thought that I would come back. In fact, the first sentence out of my husband's mouth after we touched the bronze plaque marking the southern terminus was, "We are *never* doing that again." And he meant it.

After fifty-seven days, Brew and I both learned that a supported hike is a far cry from a honeymoon or a summer vacation. Neither one of us realized how much physical and emotional support would be demanded of Brew. His hiking and tourist activities took a backseat to navigating unmarked forest service roads, searching for healthy dinner options at rural gas stations, and fielding calls from my mother.

The upshot of all this was that crewing had been so demanding for Brew that he realized it would be easier and more fun for him to transition into long-distance hiking than to continue driving support. The following summer we backpacked the 486-mile Colorado Trail together, and in 2010 we traveled to Europe and logged another 500-plus miles exploring trails in Scotland, Wales, Corsica, and the Alps.

I enjoyed hiking new paths, and despite the unavoidable conflicts that come when sharing a twenty-four-square-foot tent and feeling tethered to your partner for weeks on end, I loved hiking with my husband. But the problem remained: My last hike on the Appalachian Trail, the journey that was supposed to help me settle down and slow down, the one that was supposed to remove long-distance goal setting from my psyche, had instilled a fascination with endurance and the desire to explore my potential.

In retrospect, I was frustrated with myself for limiting my miles on the basis of sunlight and gender. I knew I could do the trail in less time and I wanted to know how much less. Five days? Seven? What about ten? Better still, could I compete for the men's record?

It also became clear to me that beyond the picturesque wildflowers of the Rocky Mountains or the thrill of summiting a Colorado Fourteener, more than the striking views of the Mont Blanc Massif or the tasty fish and chips along the coastal path in Wales, there would never be another trail like the Appalachian Trail. I missed the biodiversity and the eccentric trail community. I missed the grassy balds of the Blue Ridge Mountains and the vertical scrambles in New England. I missed the rocks and roots. I missed *my* roots. I love to travel and explore, but the Appalachian Trail will *always* be where my soul feels at home, where even in motion it feels at rest.

I wanted to know what my best was, on the trail that I loved the most. And if I didn't try, I knew I would always live with that regret.

But I also knew that going back was not solely my decision. Brew came first, the trail came second, and I would only try for the overall fastest known time if I had my husband's full support.

When I asked Brew if he would be willing to support me if I went back to attempt the overall record, he said, "If you're asking me do I *want* to help you down the trail again, do I *want* to give up another summer vacation to live out of a car and feel like every day is an opportunity for me to screw up or let you down, the answer is NO. That is not what I *want* to do."

That's that, I thought. There would be no trail record without Brew.

Then with a daring grin he looked up and said, "But . . . if this is really important to you, then you know I'm going to be behind you 100 percent."

We started making plans.

One of the first things I did was ask Warren and Horton if they would help. They both said yes. The fact that I crossed paths with Warren and Horton—even Andrew Thompson—on my first AT hike suddenly felt predestined. They were just as important to the direction of my journey as the white blazes that marked the trail.

When I asked Warren and Horton if they would support me on the trail, I also asked whether they thought I could set the overall record.

Warren said yes. And I am convinced that he meant it.

David said yes. And I believed him. Only later did Andrew Thompson divulge that Horton told him not to worry about my breaking the record. I don't necessarily think David was lying or trying to appease either one of us; he thought I *could* set the record but didn't think I *would*. And that's exactly how I felt, too.

I started my training. Day after day, mile after mile, I put in fifty-, seventy-, one-hundred-mile weeks. I would get up early and run around the neighborhood. During my lunch break I practiced yoga and later that afternoon I ate at my desk. When Brew got home from school, we would go for another run or cross-train by playing tennis, shooting some hoops, or mowing the lawn (which *is* great cross-training, by the way). As much as I could be in motion, I was to be in motion.

I needed to run during the week because of time limitations, but on the weekends, I chose to hike.

In the dark early morning hours of any given Saturday, when the rest of the world was still reveling in the glow and buzz of a Friday night, I would weigh my backpack down with firewood and gallons of water before driving to trails with the most elevation gain near Asheville. I wanted to feel heavy. I *wanted* the lactic acid to build up, to tax my muscles as much as possible through resistance and elevation to the point where when I took my pack off at the end of the day it would feel as if I were floating. That's how I wanted to feel that summer. By swapping my training weight for a daypack, I hoped I could levitate down the trail.

I tried to forgo showers and reduce my sleep to adjust my comfort level to the realities of a trail record, but Brew was not overly fond of that specific training technique and, frankly, neither was I.

When it came to my diet, I made an effort to limit processed food and eat as much protein, fruits, vegetables, and whole grains as possible. I was trying to fortify my body with whole foods, knowing that once I started hiking I would attempt to maintain a baseline of nutrition while simultaneously unwrapping countless energy bars and fast food sandwiches plus increasing my sugar and caffeine intake to higher levels than at any other season in my life.

I hated telling people that I was going to try to set the overall record. I tried to keep our plans quiet. But the absurdity and audacity of my intentions caused the news to ripple through our community like a rock thrown into a still lake. In person, most of the hikers and runners I knew at least *acted* interested, if not supportive. In the cyber world, though, where people are less polite, the responses suggested that I was egocentric for thinking I could compete with the men and I was whoring out the purity of a thru hike by trying for a record.

I was incredulous about the people who implied that I couldn't possibly love the trail and try for a record at the same time. *I* knew that I loved the trail. But I also knew if people couldn't understand that that was my primary motivation for attempting the record, then I wouldn't be able to convince them otherwise.

On the other hand, the naysayers who claimed I was unable to set the record were likely to be correct. I knew that I would most likely *not* set the record. However, unlike the haters and online trolls, I felt strongly that the likelihood of my impending failure was not based on my sex or my lack of speed. The reality is that when you are attempting to hike close to fifty miles a day for nearly fifty days straight, something's going to go wrong.

I worried about experiencing bad weather in the White Mountains or breaking my ankle on rocky terrain in Pennsylvania. I worried about contracting Lyme disease in the Mid-Atlantic or getting caught up in a yellow jacket nest and going into anaphylaxis. I was worried that Brew, like J.B., would blow five tires as he drove to a trailhead. Or worse, that he would get hurt in a car accident rushing through some unknown town trying to find me on the trail. There were countless uncontrollable factors, and the slightest dose of misfortune would mean the end of the record attempt.

Not living up to expectations is hard, regardless of whose they are or how old you are. When I was a teen, I went to a private high school where I felt constant pressure to do more and be more. For three years I bought in, giving everything I could to please other people and feed a system that I didn't feel fully invested in or recognized by. Then the summer before my senior year—weeks, in fact, before I was to begin my role as head of the school's vaunted Honor Council, senior prefect, and leading female athlete—I unenrolled.

I left prep school, stopped worrying about my college applications, and started attending the public school in my hometown. One of the faculty members at the private school told me—a seventeen year old—that I was "throwing away my future." But for the first time in four years, I wasn't miserable. Learning that I could walk away from societal expectations to become healthier and happier was a powerful lesson for a Type A teenager.

When the doctor told Scott Williamson that he couldn't hike with Achilles tendonitis after he had just taken a bus ride home through the L.A. riots, he said, "Screw it." And he went back to the trail. When Baxter State Park told Warren that he couldn't hike Katahdin in winter, he went up anyway. Ten months after the doctor told David that he might have to amputate his leg, he won a one-hundred-mile race. There are a lot of similarities that tie together record setters, but I think one of the biggest traits we have in common is that all of us somewhere deep down have a little bit of "screw it" in us. Andrew's version starts with the letter F.

Still, studies suggest that the idea of risk and failure can be paralyzing, particularly for women. In order to move past the fear of failure and the moments of doubt, I constantly asked, and then answered, these two questions:

1. What's worse: failure or regret? Regret.
2. What's the worst-case scenario of my trying for a record? I'll spend time on a trail that I love, with the man that I love, doing what I love.

When I wrestled with my bedsheets instead of sleeping, I would utter those call and response questions as if they were a Rosary prayer and then I would conclude by saying: "I belong."

I repeated my mantra standing on top of Katahdin next to the weathered brown sign that marked the path's northern terminus. It was much easier to believe now that I was actually on the trail.

In the beginning, I felt at home and at ease, even as my body adjusted to the back-to-back-to-back forty- and fifty-mile days. But I knew enough about the AT and FKTs to wonder not so much *if* something would go wrong, but when.

It took five days. Five days before my lower legs felt as if someone were scraping muscle away from bone with a knife. I had never had shin splints before and I haven't had them since, but they left me with a fear of pain that I didn't have before that summer. I never want to feel hurt that consuming again. To stub my toe was to send daggers into my shins and shock waves through my body. Going uphill was excruciating, but going downhill was unbearable. There were times when I would plant my foot and my leg would involuntarily buckle from the pain. It was as if my lower half were saying, "Nope. We're not going along with this."

I howled and yelped aloud as I hiked down the trail. I also wept. My hiking poles became crutches and ibuprofen was like a customary breath mint after every meal. In the darkness of my tent, as exhausted as I was, I spent precious minutes, even hours, elevating and icing my legs at night and wrapping them the next morning, forced into choosing first aid over sleep.

The primary treatment for shin splints is rest, but I knew that David had exited the Smokies with shin splints and run through the pain until it finally subsided. His example gave me hope, and I convinced myself that my legs would feel better in Vermont. (The upside of life-sucking mud is that it is a pillow for your feet; the soft tread would allow my legs to heal.) I rationalized that if I could make it through New Hampshire, if I could just get past the toughest mountains and the rockiest terrain, then when I crossed into the Green Mountains everything would be okay.

First, however, I had to survive the exposed ridges and extreme weather of the White Mountains. As I left the parking lot at Pinkham Notch and paralleled the base of the Presidential Range, I could see the skies darkening and feel the temperature drop. My mind went to

Andrew beating against the winter weather and being forced to bail on his second attempt at Mount Washington. My chest grew tight and my stomach felt queasy. When I reached the tree line, the wind forced me to look down. Even if I had been able to keep my head up, the route was obscured by billowing cloud cover that only occasionally offered a glimpse of the next cairn, as if it were a lighthouse guiding the way.

The limited visibility caused me to take a wrong turn, and I lost six grueling miles to the mountain and the weather. When I finally reached Crawford Notch on the far side of the Presidential Range, the rain was pouring down. I was cold, wet, and trying to do anything I could—including singing out loud—to keep my morale from completely washing away.

I told myself that the weather would change. It always does. This was the end of June; the bleak weather could not last forever. I sloshed through puddles to reach Zealand Falls. Then, though my hands felt like frozen lamb shanks, I used them to scramble up the boulders that lined the ascent to Garfield Ridge. On the crest the treadway was composed of butterlike clay and slick rocks. I couldn't maintain my footing or find much traction. I fell again and again. My legs were stiff, swollen pillars covered in red scrapes and blue and black splotches. I came out of the forest to traverse Franconia Ridge. And it was there that the weather finally changed.

On June 24, I was in the midst of a whipping sleet storm.

There was no one else on the ridge and I wasn't thinking about the record. All I could do was focus on getting down the mountain to Brew. My body was rigid, my teeth were clenched, and my fingers didn't exist. My waterproof layer was sealing the cold, wet fleece and long johns to my skin like plastic wrap. I was starving but I doubted I could open my pack or unwrap an energy bar with my numb, sock-covered hands. I also didn't want to risk stopping to grab a snack from my pack for fear that I might not start moving again.

When I finally stumbled to the base of the mountain, I was no better off. Brew assumed there had been bad weather, and he hiked in as far as he could and found a flat spot to set up the tent. When I saw it I fell inside. He helped me undress and then put me inside two sleeping bags. I kept shivering in my cocoon for a full thirty minutes until I finally had the dexterity to hold food in my hands and lift it to my lips. In the next twenty minutes, I consumed over three thousand calories.

When I couldn't eat any more, I knew I needed to get going. It was now or never. If I didn't want the record attempt to be over, I needed to get upright again and try to start hiking. I changed into the warm, dry clothes that Brew had packed in, but I couldn't find a dry pair of pants.

I looked at Brew and pointed at his lower half.

Brew looked down at his pants and then looked back up at me.

"Say please," he said.

A few minutes later, I crawled out of the tent and slowly kept moving in my husband's rain pants. Brew packed up our shelter and gear and then walked a half mile back to the road wearing boxers with the Grinch who stole Christmas on them (a strange choice for our summer hiking trip).

I kept going after the sleet storm but never fully recovered. Two days later I didn't think I could take another step. I felt overwhelmed with fatigue and fever, my body was swollen from water retention, and I couldn't sweat or pee. My systems were no longer self-regulating and my body was shutting down. Then my stomach started to churn.

For a while I was covering more ground laterally by dodging off trail into the bushes than I was progressing forward. I ran out of toilet paper and plucked striped maple leaves from the forest as voraciously as a late summer hiker gathers blueberries. Finally, I came dragging out of the forest in a wobbling, tearful haze and told Brew, "We're done. I'm done. Let's go home."

I told him how sick I was and how much I hurt. My husband is kind and sympathetic. He also, as I've mentioned, does not enjoy spending his summer days running my errands and spending nights in a tent by a trailhead. I knew he would comfort me then take me home.

But that's not what he did. "If you really want to quit," he said, "that's fine."

And I was nodding. Then he continued, "*But* . . . you can't quit right now."

I looked up at him, stupefied. I was so exhausted that I wasn't sure what he meant.

"Right now you feel too bad to make a good decision," he said. "Right now you need to eat, drink, and take medicine, then keep going a little farther, at least until tomorrow night. Then, if you still want to quit, I'll take you home."

Brew traded out my gear, loaded me down with Pepto-Bismol, then drove off. It's really hard to quit when you don't have a ride.

By the end of the day, I started to feel a little better. Even with that improvement I still felt worse than I had in my entire life. I knew that I couldn't set the record, but I realized that if I wanted to I could at least keep going.

After a day and a half, my husband didn't ask if I wanted to quit and I didn't mention anything more about stopping. We just went about our camp chores as usual, and after five hours of sleep I got dressed, wrapped my legs, downed an energy bar, and kept hiking. I didn't think I could set the record and it didn't matter. I wasn't out here to be the best; I was out here to find *my* best.

After 46 days, 11 hours, and 20 minutes I once again touched the bronze plaque atop Springer Mountain in Georgia. And once again Brew, who was right there with me, said, "We are *never* doing that again." There would never be a need.

We had set the overall record. But more important, I had found something deep within me that I thought might be there, though I couldn't be convinced until I was put to the test.

Now, I had my answer. My body and mind confirmed that I had left everything on the trail. The moment it all ended, I didn't think I had the strength to wobble the nine-tenths of a mile from Springer's summit to the nearby parking lot.

It had taken letting go of the record to put it within reach. Once I shifted my focus away from fastest known times and miles per hour and Andrew Thompson's itinerary, I felt less pressure and more joy. And as a result, my daily miles quickly increased. Even when Warren Doyle and David Horton came to the trail to help us out, I quickly realized that I couldn't always do what they asked of me. I wasn't going to set the record the same way they had. I couldn't subsist on three hours of sleep a night as Warren suggested, nor could I run the trail as David goaded me to do. I weighed their wisdom and accepted much of their advice, but ultimately, if I was to make it to the end, I had to listen to my body, find my *own* pace, and take ownership of the everyday decisions.

I learned that endurance, even amid a competition, is still an individual journey. Everyone takes part in a unique struggle, and at some point, you will need to unlock your own secrets in order to keep going.

In my mind, the experience is not organized chronologically by day or systematically arranged by location. Instead, the record is an abstract collage of memorable views and emotions. It is the drowning sound of my heartbeat in my eardrums as I ascended mountains in the dark and the abrasive feel of sediment lodged in my socks after slogging through a rain shower or river crossing. The experience of setting the record was captured in the reaction of my husband at each road crossing.

Still, some suggest that I didn't fully experience or "take in" the trail while hiking forty-seven miles per day. The truth is I have never felt more present. A recreational hike allows you to zone out; a record forces you to focus. Whether it was excruciating or exhilarating didn't matter; in the end, I felt every step.

If I had to summarize the journey succinctly, it would be through an exchange I shared with another thru hiker in Pennsylvania. We had started walking together in the midday July heat and continued leapfrogging each other on the rock-strewn ledges of the state's coal region long after the sun had set.

At one point the gangly backpacker turned to me, spotlighting my face with his glaring headlamp. The strong beam forced my eyes sideways, away from the rocks. I took a slight stumble but did not fall.

He kept his interrogation light trained on me as I regained my balance, then asked, more critically than inquisitively, "Are you even having fun out here?"

I stopped and lifted my head toward him for a minute, meeting his spotlight with my own penetrating beam.

"No," I said. "No, I'm not having fun. But I think this might be better than fun."

I turned my face back toward the rocks, then looked up to orient myself with the next white blaze. I put one foot in front of the other and continued down the trail. My companion paused for a second or two, then continued tailing me. Quietly.

When I finished the Appalachian Trail, Brew and I were inundated with questions. Everyone wanted to know how many pairs of shoes I'd gone through and the number of bears I had seen. They asked how much weight I'd lost, how much sleep I'd gotten, and how many hours I'd hiked each day. I rattled off the answers: seven shoes, thirty-six bears, fifteen pounds, five or six hours of sleep, eighteen hours of walking. But as with a box score in a game of basketball or baseball, the statistics of a record are just numbers on a page; they will never tell the full story of a trail record. And as I mentioned earlier, everyone wanted to know, "What's next?"

I didn't have an answer for them then, but in hindsight I wish that I had politely replied, "That was enough."

I also answered dozens of questions about gender.

In many ways, it felt as if gender disappeared on the trail. As the journey progressed, I stopped seeing the fastest known time as a competition between men and women. In so doing, I quit thinking that I was at an advantage or disadvantage because of my sex and I truly did start to believe that I belonged. I went from merely *telling* myself that I was on an equal playing field with the record setters of the past to actually believing that it was true. And yet, being a woman underlay much of my motivation and thought process.

The same transformation I had experienced as a twenty-one-year-old when I realized I was a part of nature—a part of all that beauty—was intensified. I felt I was also tapping into something primal that said I am beautiful *because I endure.*

One of the determining factors in trying for the record was that going forward I knew I wanted to be a mom, and looking back I didn't want to have questions about what my body could do on the trail. On the trail, I constantly compared the experience to bearing a child. I theorized that the weight of a pack was no different from the weight of pregnancy and the pain I experienced might be comparable to delivery. (If someone had offered me an epidural during my bout of shin splints, I would have accepted it.) I felt confident the energy reserves I needed to finish the trail were there because my body was programmed to prioritize not *my* needs but my ability to reproduce. As a woman, I always had something left to give.

In fact, at one point, when I was thinking through the evolutionary edge of childbearing at a time when I felt severely fatigued, nauseated, and short of breath, it occurred to me that I needed to rule out pregnancy as the cause of my symptoms.

I hadn't had my period since starting the trail, which didn't come as a surprise, since women often become irregular or go without a cycle due to high levels of stress or physical exertion. But I started to worry that perhaps oral birth control was not effective when paired with fifty miles and upward of seven thousand calories a day. At a minimum, I doubted that the pharmaceutical companies had performed *that* product testing.

Horton was driving out to see us that morning, so I asked him to pick up a pregnancy test for me on his way. When the result came back negative, I kept hiking. I was relieved to not be pregnant—yet. (I was also flattered and entertained by the thought of Horton buying a pregnancy test for me.)

In case it's not clear from the preceding anecdote, I *needed* Brew that summer. He was my complement. I felt deeply attracted to those attributes he had that I didn't possess. Some of that had to do with personality and part of it was tied to his masculinity. All I know is that by combining our differences, I accomplished something I never could have achieved as an individual.

When I say that gender seemed to disappear on the trail, perhaps what I am trying to convey is that gender limitations disappeared. And maybe that is the best definition of feminism I can offer, to be able to embrace your gender identity without societal or self-imposed limitations.

Now when I get asked if men or women hold an advantage in endurance sports, I take a line from my good friend Horton and respond, "Both." Endurance is both individual and universal. Many of my motives in setting the record were feminine, and they helped me uncover my human ability to endure.

FKTs are not like most sports in which you try to add muscle or acquire new skills. In order to excel at endurance, you have to peel away the layers to discover what's already there. You leave behind your level of comfort and your physical—and emotional—weight, you let go of public perception and mental limitations, you go beyond your age and your gender, and beneath all that there is something raw that connects us all.

Once I set the FKT, I was a stronger, more outspoken feminist. I was finally at the point where I believed that my ability was of equal value, and it took feeling like an equal for me to realize that I wasn't always being treated like one. I had to walk more than ten thousand miles and set a record to dispel the gender bias I had accepted—the one that society, media, and the marketplace present, overtly and subconsciously, on a daily basis. And I'm determined not to make my daughter go that far to claim her full self-worth.

Now I know that, as an individual and as a woman, I can do much more than what my community expects, what my society allows, and even more than what I think is possible.

So then why do I feel as if I am doing less? I have to remind myself these days that endurance is not always about movement. Sometimes the only way to endure is to stay put.

I am not setting records and I am not making progress in a literal sense, but I am doing what I want to do—what I chose to do. Five years after setting the record, I have come to accept that the legacy of setting a fastest known time is not having your name listed in the annals of record setters, but in the application of endurance to everyday occurrences. When life feels hopeless, or unfair, or completely out of my control, I remember the new opportunities, experiences, and encounters that arise when you are willing to take one more step.

I think about the FKT when my daughter's internal alarm clock goes off at the same time I used to crawl out of my tent to start hiking: 4:45 a.m. The early start gives us time to get her dressed in an outfit of her choosing (that doesn't match) and make her a breakfast (that she refuses to eat) before walking her to preschool. (Don't worry, it's not that far.)

Then, the work day starts and I need to respond to emails, hop on a conference call, settle a personnel issue that popped up at the hiking company, and pack for an upcoming work trip—all while a writing deadline looms. I take a break midway through to send my brother a birthday card that will arrive five days late. And have I mentioned that our lawn *always* needs to be mowed?

I try *not* to think about my FKT when I am out sucking wind on my standard three-mile run around the neighborhood, wondering whether I'll be able to finish the loop without peeing on myself. (Thank you, motherhood.)

At night, Brew and I work together to set out on the dining table the dinner he has picked up. Then we divide the bedtime routine of reading books, brushing teeth, and checking under the bed for trolls. When it's finally just the two of us, we disagree about whose turn it is to do the dishes or who forgot to pay our overdue bill. Our argument is cut short by a little girl with a bad dream. So we go into her bedroom and we all just hold each other.

And as I lie there in bed, next to my family, I once again think back to the forty-six days when the only way to move forward was to work as a team. And I remind myself that sometimes you are so consumed by the task at hand that you don't realize that you are on your way to accomplishing something amazing.

CHAPTER EIGHT

The Science of Endurance

"For the majority of human existence, exercise was the norm or the baseline and being sedentary was the exception."

—Shawn Bearden

"We're all movers—and the movement is more important than the mechanics."

—JPD

When I was a small child, I loved nothing more than visiting my grandmother, who was a retired children's librarian. I would curl up next to her on her green velvet couch that smelled of floral potpourri and she would read Greek myths and Aesop's fables with accents and intonations that brought the stories to life in her living room.

My favorite tale was that of the tortoise and the hare. My grandmother's reading skills made the legendary duel sound as exciting as a live radio broadcast of game seven in the World Series. I was on the edge of my seat willing the turtle to touch the finisher's tape first. And when that happened, I launched off the couch and jumped up and down cheering. (I was very young and it was hard to sit still. Nonetheless, the librarian in my grandmother did not appreciate the loud response.)

Now when I read the same timeless classic to my daughter, I try to bring in the level of suspense that my grandmother captured, but because of my experience with trail records I am also inclined to take long pauses as I try to dissect the strategy of each animal. I wonder what Aesop was really trying to tell us with this fable.

Did the rabbit lose because his heart rate was too high or because running and hopping took a greater toll on his body than walking?

Was the turtle's diet better? Was it possible to stay cooler and better hydrated with a shell?

Why did the hare need a nap? Was he just lazy or sleep deprived?

Did the turtle win with persistence or was there an underlying physiological edge that has been overlooked.

When I close the book, my daughter does not jump up and yell. Instead, she looks at me and asks, "Now can we read the book that I want?" (She's started to pick up on my attempt to indoctrinate her with endurance reads.)

The story of the tortoise and the hare has always resonated with me. One of my goals in life is to not try to outmuscle or outpace those around me, but to keep my head down and focus on what I'm doing so that I can do it well. In school, sports, and my work I have a history of being boringly good. It's not sexy, but it's effective.

On the record, I believed that consistent output over a prolonged period would be more efficient than short bursts of speed followed by lengthier rests. In other words, I wanted to hike, not run. I rationalized that walking would mean less impact on my joints, a reduced risk of falling, and decreased recovery time; it just seemed like a more natural way to cover more than two thousand miles.

Most folks would concede that walking quickly might allow one to outpace a severely fatigued runner or be more effective on a steep uphill, but logically it still makes sense that a runner would reach the finish line before a hiker, right?!

I ran my first road race when I was fourteen. It was a ten-kilometer run that wove through the streets of downtown Naples, Florida. We were there as a family for spring break and I decided that signing up for a race would offer a change from sitting beside the pool or playing board games with my brothers. I had two goals for the event. The first was that I wanted to finish. And the second was that I didn't want to walk. I also really wanted a race T-shirt—so make that three goals.

It was exhilarating to line up shoulder to shoulder with the hundreds of other participants at the starting line. When the bullhorn sounded, I kept pace with the runners around me. People were standing on the sidewalk and in front yards cheering us on. I was running a little faster than I was used to, but I didn't think anything of it. My adrenaline was pumping. Eventually, I started to notice the burning sensation in my chest and the fatigue in my legs, but I ignored them both. Even at fourteen, I knew that this was a race and that races were *supposed* to hurt.

But then the hurt became too much. The tightness in my chest made it hard to breathe and my legs started to feel like limp noodles. The people who'd been beside me were now way ahead of me. And instead of running, I was shuffling. But damn it, at least I wasn't walking. Then a spry older gentleman with a red, white, and blue headband, perfectly bronzed skin, and obscenely short shorts wriggled his lean hips past me by speed walking. It was an image I would not soon forget.

I had run throughout high school, I'd completed marathons in college, and had gotten into ultramarathons in my twenties. When I thought about tackling the record on the Appalachian Trail, I knew I'd hike as much of it as I possibly could. That may seem counterintuitive, but I had learned by then, from the bronzed Floridian to the number of ultramarathoners I saw power-hiking uphill in 50k races, that a powerful hiking stride bested a tired run-shuffle any day.

Hiking is what worked for me in the long run, but I wasn't sure that it would be the best approach for everyone. To this day, I wonder if a runner is going to come along and eclipse my record by several days. Even with all my experience, I'm still not sure what the best strategy would be. So I decided to ask a friend, ultrarunner, and scientist what he thought.

"We are *built* for walking," said Shawn Bearden, professor of exercise physiology at Idaho State University. I got to know Shawn a while ago when he interviewed me for his podcast, *Science of Ultra*.

Since 2015, he has produced dozens of conversations with the world's leading physiologists, runners, sports psychologists, cardiologists, and nutritionists on the topic of ultrarunning. In short, he knows his stuff. And now it was my turn to pick his brain.

We started chatting about walking versus running, and Shawn immediately harkened back to early man to help me understand our physical design and drive. Homo sapiens followed herds and tracked wild animals. We migrated with the seasons to find more forgiving weather or suitable grounds for foraging plants. We fled on foot to avoid threats from neighboring nomadic tribes. If we needed to get somewhere—if we wanted to live at all—conditions demanded that we spend a large part of our lives on the move.

"Historically speaking," Shawn said, "humans were active and moving 99 percent of the time. That's how we evolved and that's what our bodies expect. We have to start turning around this idea that exercise is a stimulus. For the majority of human existence, exercise was the norm or the baseline and being sedentary was the exception."

The study of human history is the study of walking *and* the study of trails. The well-beaten dirt paths that wind through our landscape are responsible for dispersing goods and ideas. Where mountains, plains, and marshes separated us, trails linked us together. And for the majority of humans, the most efficient and sustainable method for getting around was to strike your heel on the ground, roll forward on the ball of your foot, and repeat that thousands of times a day. But there are times when walking just isn't fast enough. So for both survival and 5ks, humans have developed the ability to run.

Obviously, we're all walkers, but I always believed that we were runners, too. And I was convinced that Shawn, who was currently training for a hundred-mile race, would agree. Instead, he completely downplayed my efforts to paint humans as adept runners.

"We are built to keep going, keep moving; we are built mostly for walking," said Shawn.

It turns out that our most effective evolutionary "assets" for running—our butts—are engineered more for sprinting and climbing than for long-distance races.

He continued, "The idea that our ancestors evolved to be long-distance runners is an extension of a misunderstanding of persistence hunting. Evidence suggests that the humans who tracked animals were only going about thirty kilometers or so in a hunt, and that they walked the majority of that distance. There was only a little running."

"But . . ." I stammered, and hesitated a bit before treading on sacred ground.

"Aren't we born to run?" Shawn interjected.

Before I could reply, he responded resolutely. "No. No, we have not evolved to be distance runners. We're not even really built to run a marathon. We are born to walk fast and sometimes run."

Shawn discounted the idea that Homo sapiens evolved from distance runners by defining persistence hunting—which involves chasing prey to the point of exhaustion—as a fast-paced walk with a few bursts of running.

If that strategy worked best for prehistoric man, I wondered if it would also be the best approach on a trail record. Maybe I could have completed the trail faster if I'd been willing to run the flat and downhill sections of the trail?

Shawn suggested that when covering long distances on trails, walking uphill is always the better approach. The same holds true for level ground. Running is obviously a faster way to go downhill but causes more damage. You want to move downhill as fast as possible with as little effort as possible, letting gravity do the work while you use your legs as subtle shock absorbers. So when carrying a pack—as on a self-supported or unsupported FKT—running downhill is a bad choice. Speed doesn't outweigh the ability to keep moving injury-free.

I had once heard Warren say that a hiker can push all he wants to go uphill, but he should exercise caution and travel his own pace on the downhill. He warns: "Don't try to keep up with the semi on a downhill and don't punch on the breaks."

Hikers and backpackers don't use trekking poles to look like misplaced alpine skiers but to reduce the joint pressure and inflammation in their legs and hips. For hikers and runners alike the downhill can be harder on the body than a steep climb. But it takes a larger toll on the runners.

As Shawn points out, when you walk you always have one foot on the ground. If you're running, then at some point your whole body is off the ground. Running forces you to lift your body up off the earth. The landing phase requires substantially different impact—greater impact. It also requires more energy— more calories.

Over a week or two weeks, it's not much of a problem to pound and run and use excessive calories. But for weeks on end or several months, those very little things that happen with each step start to add up. And they can make a real difference. You have to run if you want to win hundred-mile races or complete them within the cutoff times, but for a two-thousand-plus-mile FKT the strategy has to change.

What Shawn and I didn't discuss is that athletes are willing to wreck their bodies to reach the end of the trail. Scientifically speaking, walking is the more self-preserving method of covering more than two-thousand miles, but there are plenty of runners willing to sacrifice knee cartilage and future athletic aspirations for one FKT. Hikers might come out of the endeavor with less physiological damage, but that doesn't mean that a runner won't set the record.

I also need to emphasize that the topic at hand is entirely different from the modern objective of maintaining a healthy lifestyle. For 99 percent of folks, *anytime* is a great time to run. Getting out of our sedentary lifestyles and working up a sweat is healthy and important. But working up too much of a sweat on a record attempt can be a problem. This discussion is about the distance runners will travel before hikers pass them.

According to Shawn, "The two components of utmost importance when carrying your body a very long distance are wear and tear and energetics."

I wasn't sure of the exact definition of "energetics," but its root made me think that Shawn was referring to output and exertion. For a layperson I wasn't far off, but for a scientist like Shawn energetics encompasses the entire energy transfer process, including aspects such as thermodynamics.

Humans are able to walk all day because we evolved the necessary trait of regulating our body temperature with sweat. The human body's ability to stay cool during prolonged periods of exercise historically helped us track and hunt animals. Today, it helps a construction worker put in a ten-hour day in the summer sun, or a farmer work his land for hours in high humidity, or an endurance athlete set an FKT. The key to staying out there is to work steady, not hard.

"Ideally, you want to be covered with damp skin or a thin layer of sweat that is evaporating," said Shawn. "You don't want to be dripping. Sweat that drips is precious fluid wasted."

The more I talked with Shawn, the more I regretted vying for a record in the heat of the summer. The fact that I'd started in mid-June and finished in late July meant my body was having to work overtime to cool itself down, which led to a substantially higher average heart rate than if I'd been pushing myself down the trail during the cooler months.

On the other hand, summer afforded me more daylight than if I'd made a spring or fall attempt—and I didn't have to deal with snow or ice. For a particularly strong night hiker or someone with loads of experience running ultras in the dark, daylight might not matter. But as a southern girl, I was conditioned to heat, and I think opting for daylight was still the right plan of attack. If I had to do it over again I might move my start date up a few weeks, but not months.

I had never before thought about sweat as "wasted fluid." It seemed counterintuitive—or perhaps just countercultural. In America, we have a gym culture that idolizes perspiration. You hit the treadmill or pump iron hoping to work up a good sweat.

When I leave a workout dripping, I feel as if I have cleansed my pores, rid my body of toxins, and done something I can be proud of. But the stream of water running down our temples and the salt stains on our workout clothes cannot replace the benefits of a full day of motion. We cannot condense our primary identity as pedestrians into a thirty-minute workout.

I love to walk all day. And unlike most, I have been able to fulfill that desire for weeks or months at a time. But I have not been able to turn it into a full-time lifestyle. So for most of the year I'm going to go to Zumba, or Crossfit, or Pilates, or head out my front door for a run. With work and family, I can't dedicate much more than forty-five minutes a day to my personal exercise routine (and that includes the postworkout shower).

But I can start my day with a few minutes of sit-ups or push-ups. When I'm at work, I can take a break and stretch, walk around the block, or find a flight of stairs to climb. And at the end of the day, when I want nothing more than to eat a bowl of ice cream in front of a twenty-minute sitcom, I can choose to be an engaged parent and follow my daughter around the house as she plays dress-up and builds pillow forts.

In our office-dwelling, car-driving culture it's impossible for most people to sustain consistent movement throughout the day, but we can still sneak it into our routine in a way that reminds us of our body's purpose and makes us feel much healthier.

I knew that athletes and researchers alike have pointed to the benefits of a relatively low and controlled heart rate for sustained aerobic activity, and that was another of the reasons I tried to hike my way into the record books instead of run my way in.

As he did with many of the ideas I put forth, Shawn hemmed and hawed about my theory.

"There's no doubt heart rate is one indicator of how hard your body is working," he said, "but it's not necessarily an indicator of how *fast* you are moving. Other factors beyond pace can increase heart rate, including anxiety, sleep deprivation, negative mood, as well as hydration and body temperature."

It also made sense that the stress of arriving at a remote road crossing and not spotting my crew or of stumbling across a bear or venomous snake in the dark would've caused my heart rate to spike even if I were at a standstill.

"Heart rate and energy expenditure can be disconnected," Shawn said. "But typically, if you're keeping your heart rate down, you're keeping your energy output lower. Considering heart rate and wanting to keep it down is the right approach. The heart does well when it stays just above a resting level. It's very comfortable doing that for an extended period of time."

What's normal for most well-conditioned athletes can be a red flag for the average person. When I delivered our daughter years ago, the nurse had to keep coming in to check on me because my resting heart rate was low and was triggering an alarm on one of the machines.

"Are you a runner?" the nurse asked.

"I'm a *hiker*," I replied with a slight chip on my shoulder. But then I added, "I like to run, too."

She gave me a cockeyed look, readjusted my blood pressure sleeve, and walked back to the nurses' station.

Most serious athletes have low resting heart rates, but endurance athletes are seemingly just one level up from a corpse. For that reason, you would think runners would have incredible cardiovascular health. But David Horton had to undergo septuple bypass heart surgery despite logging more than one hundred thousand miles in his lifetime. And there are stories of well-trained marathoners and ultra-marathoners dropping dead from heart attacks.

Toward the end of my FKT, there were a few times when I felt an intense ache in my chest. It never lasted more than a few minutes, but when it happened, it hurt—and it scared me. I'd never had chest pain before. I could typically walk through it or "walk it out," just as I did with everything else. But on the last night of my AT record, I was hiking uphill with a friend pacing me a few feet ahead. It was close to midnight and I'd been on the move for nearly twenty hours when I started to feel the tightness in my chest. As I kept walking it became more difficult to breathe.

"I need . . . to . . . I need to . . . stop," I panted.

I crouched like a catcher in baseball and put my head between my knees. It felt as if I had a cramp in my torso that was making its way from my heart to my lungs and up my windpipe, constricting everything as it went along. Trying to take a deep breath was like sipping a scalding-hot cup of tea. Tears ran down my cheeks. My friend knelt behind me massaging my shoulders and imploring me to take long, slow breaths.

The night air was filled with the sound of crickets, north Georgia barn owls, and my labored, wheezing breath. After a few minutes of crying and gasping for air, my inhalations became deeper and longer. As my chest filled with air, I could feel the flexibility and energy return to my limbs. I wiped my eyes with a dirt-covered forearm, unfurled from my stance like a fern frond, and nodded to let my friend know we could start hiking.

After my trail record, I worried that the stresses of it might have done permanent damage to my heart. So after my daughter was born, I decided to visit a cardiologist and find out. I had an echocardiogram and took a stress test and then I waited nervously for the results.

A few days later, I was hiking when I noticed I'd missed a call from my doctor. I pushed the play button on my phone and listened to the voicemail. "Don't worry," said the doctor, "you have a *beautiful* heart."

When I told Shawn about the chest pains I'd experienced, he said, "It might have been a case of costochondritis. That's basically an aching in your rib cage. It's a common condition in athletes. There is no evidence today that endurance or extreme endurance pursuits cause any long-term damage to the heart."

Shawn explained that what we've heard in recent news stories and in studies in which people have died from heart attacks during endurance exercise involved people who already had disease before they got into endurance sports. They started doing endurance because they were smokers and overweight and wanted to change their lives. They came in with some weakening of the heart muscle to begin with.

Shawn assuaged my fears and convinced me that extreme endurance is not going to create any long-term health problems that weren't already underlying issues. And with that, the pendulum swung and I wondered if prolonged exercise resulted in any health benefits.

"My gut reaction," said Shawn, "is that there aren't any benefits to running or hiking fast over long distances versus moderate, sustained exercise."

I was admittedly a little surprised. I hoped that a trail record might somehow be good for my health. I could even accept that it might have some negative ramifications. But I found it hard to believe that something so extreme could ultimately be a neutral endeavor.

In 2011, I walked my way to a trail record. And only once on my forty-six-day push did someone pass me. It happened one morning along the banks of the Potomac River as I followed the Chesapeake and Ohio Canal Towpath, one of the few places along the two-thousand-plus-mile trail where the tread resembles an urban greenway more than an amalgamation of jumbled roots and rocks.

I was cruising along at close to four miles an hour when a woman in a cobalt blue wind suit whom I assumed to be in her early seventies skirted past me in a steady jog. She was going just *slightly* faster than

I was. As much as I tried to keep pace with her, I could hear her synthetic outfit swishing out of earshot and see her incandescent silhouette shrink to the size of a Smurf, then disappear.

I let out a little laugh when I think of a strong, fierce, record-setting hiker striding her way down the towpath only to have a wind-suit-wearing grandma swish by in a steady jog. The same thing happens when I think back to being a young, fit high school student who thought she was running when a sun-kissed Floridian in a headband waddled past her.

When I think about the people who might be able to surpass current trail records, runners and hikers both come to mind. Fast is fast, endurance is endurance. Perhaps athletes get too hung up on identifying themselves as either hikers or runners? Perhaps we all get too caught up in which category of exercise we ascribe to. At the end of the day, we're all just movers—and the movement is more important than the mechanics.

There are a number of factors that can affect performance and recovery time. Gait, heart rate, and thermoregulation are a few of the big ones, but on my record attempt, I also wondered to what extent age, sleep, and nutrition affected a person's performance.

When David Horton started his Pacific Crest Trail record attempt at 5:55 a.m. on June 5, he was fifty-five years old.

"Did you think you were at a disadvantage because of your age?"

"No," he said. "Looking back now, maybe I was, but at the time I didn't think so."

"But you set the AT record when you were forty-one years old. Didn't it feel different physically to set a record fourteen years later?"

"No, nothing felt different," he responded. "I recovered just as well during the PCT record when I was fifty-five as I did on the AT when I was forty-one. I also trained just as hard at fifty-five."

It was hard to believe that there was little difference in his record attempts, and I kept probing for some distinctions.

"Did it take longer to recover when it was all over?" I asked.

"Not really. I never thought about being old. Looking back, I think maybe I just didn't try to go fast enough. The record's been lowered several times since then." (With that, Horton pinpointed a similarity between all former record holders. Once our hard-earned mark is surpassed, we all think that we should have gone a little faster.)

The FKT on the Appalachian Trail had a head start when compared with records on the Pacific Crest Trail. At the turn of the twenty-first century, the bar had already been set pretty high in the East, which was probably the result of being "the" trail for decades on end, not to mention meandering through the country's most densely populated region.

In high-profile American sports there's a concept called "East Coast bias," according to which reporters focus more on the teams in the eastern region of the United States because game times line up TV viewership and readership is naturally more interested in what's going on locally than on the other side of the country, where there are fewer fans and teams.

In recent years, a "West Coast bias" seems to have emerged in outdoor sports, placing greater emphasis on what happens in, say, the Rockies and the Sierras than in the Blue Ridge Mountains or the Adirondacks. Renowned downhill skiers have migrated from slopes in Vermont and New Hampshire to Utah, Colorado, and British Columbia. Rock climbers have flocked to Yosemite and Joshua Tree. Elite trail runners have done the same, and this has led to a growing interest in FKTs on the far side of the western continental divide. This tendency in outdoor sports over the past few decades has loosely paralleled prospectors heading west during the California Gold Rush. Between 2005 and 2016 the supported record on the Pacific Crest Trail has been lowered by a span of nearly two weeks. During that same period, the AT record has been lowered by only two days.

In 2014, a twenty-one-year-old cross-country runner from

Boston College named Joe McConaughy headed west with some buddies and lowered the supported FKT on the Pacific Crest Trail to fifty-three days, which comes out to an astounding fifty miles a day.

"I was really surprised at that," Horton said. "Joe was so young and inexperienced. All he'd done was run cross-country in college."

I didn't find it any more shocking that a twenty-one-year-old set the record than that Horton did it at age fifty-five. I figured they were both outliers and exceptions. It seemed to me that the perfect age for endurance might fall smack in the middle. But when I asked Shawn about this, his response surprised me.

"There's no ideal age for endurance," he said. "There are biological and physiological changes that would favor endurance and there are others that would work against it. For example, some cardiovascular declines might impair performance but at the same time there are adjustments happening in our muscles that are beneficial for long-distance events. There might be an ideal age for each person, but that can vary tremendously based on the individual."

I was twenty-eight when I set the overall record on the Appalachian Trail. Warren was with Brew and me for the first twelve days of that record attempt. On multiple occasions he said, "Genius is wisdom and youth." The statement was a bit cryptic, but I was pretty sure I knew what he meant: He was the wisdom and I was the youth.

There were fleeting moments when it seemed our partnership reached an ethereal level, but often his wisdom and my youth were at odds. We frequently disagreed on how far I should hike in a given day. He always wanted me to go a little farther, not necessarily to hike faster so much as just to sleep less.

"Sleep is an emotional need," he would say.

After being sleep-deprived for twelve straight days and hiking through shin splints and bad weather in New Hampshire, I found that sleep did not feel as much like an emotional need as a physical necessity. My body ached, my legs were swollen and inflamed, my decision making was impaired, and I figured if I didn't start getting at least six hours of sleep a night to rest my legs and my brain, I'd have a snowball's chance in hell of continuing, let alone setting any kind of record. I was convinced that diving deeper into the sleep deprivation would result in either a serious physical injury or an egregious mental mistake.

Looking back, I think Warren was right. Maybe that's because I have more experience—more wisdom—now. I know that I've referenced the birth of my daughter nearly as much as my FKT, but that's because they're both life changing, completely stressful, and entirely worthwhile, and they share a similar skill set. So . . . after the birth of our daughter, I spent a solid three months longing for meaningful REM sleep and feeling grateful whenever our baby slept more than two straight hours. Somehow, I survived and so did she.

I knew of Warren's eccentric sleep patterns—that he would often drive ten plus hours through the night to get home after a contra dance in Pennsylvania or Connecticut, or he would sleep in his car in a McDonald's parking lot or a Wal-Mart off I-81. But I was surprised when I started asking other FKTers how much shut-eye they required and found out they'd all needed less sleep on their record attempts than I did.

"You know what really pissed me off?" Andrew Thompson asked.

I could imagine quite a few things that would piss Andrew off.

"The fact that I was only getting five hours of sleep a night and that half the time I'd wake up and find myself lying half-naked in leaves and dirt outside my tent. I was so tired that when I'd wake up in the middle of the night to take a leak, I'd unzip my tent, do my business, then never fully make it back inside. My alarm would go off and I'd be all stiff and cold from sleeping on the forest floor. And I'd still be picking sticks out of my hair into the late morning and early afternoon. I was only getting a couple hours' sleep a night and the sleep wasn't even that *good*. I mean, c'mon. Really?"

I laughed. Fortunately, I'd never woken up outside my tent after a midnight pee break. But one time I did wake up inside the tent with Brew shaking me frantically.

"What are you doing?" he whispered urgently.

I mumbled something under my breath and he said, "What?!"

Then I spoke up and pleaded anxiously, "I can't find the trail . . . I've gotta keep *hiking*."

"It's not time to hike yet," he said. "It's the middle of the night. Go back to bed."

I heard what he was saying, but even as I answered him I was still in a fog, not fully aware that I was up on my knees inside my sleeping bag leaning against the tent's nylon sidewall, both hands grasping for the zipper to the outside. In my dream, I was night hiking and had gotten desperately lost. My mind was racing. All I could think about was the time I'd wasted and the miles I needed to make up.

I'm sure that if I had gotten out of the tent, I would've started sleepwalking through the forest and gotten lost without a headlamp or reference points. (From that point on Brew slept with one eye open. And if I *did* wake up in the middle of the night to pee, he would stir and stay awake until I made it safely back to our tent.)

When I was chasing that record, I spent a large part of my waking hours fantasizing about sleep. I wanted it more than I wanted anything—more than fresh produce or a home-cooked meal, more than a cold beer or a glass of wine, more even than a hot shower or a soak in the tub. The one bargain I made with myself during the record attempt was that if I could keep going and make it to Springer Mountain, for the rest of my life I could sleep whenever I wanted and for as long as I wanted. And nothing would be taboo. I could take naps in the middle of the workday or indulge in consistent ten-hour nights on our memory foam mattress. Admittedly, my pledge went out the window as soon as I made it to Springer Mountain, but it helped me reach the finish.

Now that I had the opportunity to bend the ear of an expert, I knew exactly what I wanted to ask.

"Shawn," I said, "when it comes to physical performance and endurance, is sleep an emotional need, or a physical one?"

Without hesitation or qualification, Shawn said, "It is 100 percent emotional."

Damn it, Warren! That was *not* the answer I wanted to hear.

Shawn felt sure that sleep is not necessary for physical recovery, it is a brain need, but one the brain will make a priority during a multiweek or multimonth endurance pursuit.

I went on to discover that the primary reason for sleep is not to restore our body, but to restore our brain. If we want our body to recover, we need to stop moving, not sleep. In other words, sitting down will help your weary body as much as a nap will.

The catch is that when we get tired, our brain likes to play tricks and spread lies. We've already covered the angle of hallucinations, but the mind also likes to tell the body that it needs to sleep even when it doesn't. Our mind can increase our perceived level of exertion, and a task will seem more challenging and exhausting than it really is. The brain is trying to force the body to give it what it needs. Sneaky brain! But our bodies can play a little trick of their own by resetting the perceived level of exertion with a ten- or fifteen-minute catnap.

I thought back to Captain Barclay, the famous British Pedestrian who walked a thousand miles in a thousand hours. During his successful feat, he walked one mile per hour—as dictated—and often snacked and took a ten-minute snooze before starting up again. In thirty-eight days, he never slept more than thirty minutes at a stretch.

I hate to admit it now, but there were a few blissful nights on my record attempt when I got seven hours of sleep. I feel like such a lush saying that! I should also point out that there were several occasions when I only slept three or four hours. It would be interesting to see an FKT attempt by someone who intended to get his or her rest in small increments, rather than clumping it all together at night.

To stay awake and alert, I usually had one or at most two caffeinated drinks a day. Usually Brew would bring me coffee from a gas station in the morning. The brown liquid wasn't for taste or pleasure, it was merely a vehicle for cream, sugar, and caffeine. By midafternoon I might take a few swigs from a can of Pepsi or Coke from our SUV to help wash down my turkey and cheese sandwich or whatever I was eating for my second lunch. That's right, I typically had a second lunch. And a second breakfast. And a second dinner. I was in full-on Hobbit mode. My job was to get as many calories in as I could in ten to fifteen minutes while Brew reorganized my pack and filled it with snacks and other items that I would need for the upcoming stretch.

I typically wouldn't go more than an hour and a half without eating something. If you want to hike fifty miles a day, you've got to have fuel. I tried to consume upward of seven thousand calories a day, and it never felt like enough. By the time I set the record, I'd lost fifteen pounds and I positively *abhorred* chewing. Those final few weeks I kept asking Brew to find me food that I could swallow without chewing—things like high-protein energy drinks, milkshakes, and fruit smoothies.

Diet is another variable that each FKTer has his or her own take on. In 2006, Warren hiked the John Muir Trail in two weeks on a diet that consisted exclusively of Little Debbies. And here's the kicker — Warren *lost* weight along the way.

While David Horton's diet is a step up from Warren's, on any given day I would almost be guaranteed to find double-stuffed Oreos, neon-orange Cheetos, and luminescent diet Sunkist in his pantry or pack.

"I try to eat relatively healthy off trail," David said without a hint of irony. "On the trail, it's a matter of getting enough energy or at least getting as much as you can. We'd try to find pig bars near the trail."

"Sorry, pig bars?" I interjected.

"You know," he said, "all-you-can-eat buffets. I could go there and eat as much as I wanted, load up on calories, and not waste much time. There are times on a record when you don't want to eat. But you *have* to. I'm always glad when I reach the end because I can eat whatever I want whenever I want."

When I visited Scott Williamson at his home in Truckee, California, he put out a carton of organic strawberries to complement the birdseed that he'd distributed for the Steller's jays that dive-bombed his deck. "The carton says they're organic, but to me they smell like some type of chemical or spray," he said. A frugal hiker had just donated a six-dollar carton of organic strawberries to the birds because they didn't smell right.

Scott said, "I try to eat a mostly whole-foods-based and mostly organic diet as much as it's possible and practical. More so at home than on the trail, but as much as I can on the trail, too. I am not a vegan nor am I a vegetarian, although I was on a vegan and sometimes raw vegan diet throughout most of the first ten years that I hiked long distances."

He continued, "My on-trail diet tends to be pretty repetitive. Breakfast, lunch, and snacks consist of homemade energy bars, beef jerky, some type of trail mix, whole grain fig bars, peanut butter, usually some kind of sweet like a natural licorice bar, and maybe a commercial protein bar. For dinner, I almost always eat dehydrated refried beans with corn chips and add olive oil liberally. I don't generally carry a stove on my summer hikes. I prefer to cold soak my dinners to avoid cooking, partly to save weight and time and partly as a result of the explosive fire conditions we have throughout the West every summer."

Knowing that dietary approaches among endurance athletes varied from raw veganism to Little Debbie, I was interested to hear Shawn's thoughts on nutrition.

"When you're covering such great distance, whether you're running or walking and whether it's supported or unsupported, you're burning *way* too many calories to worry about the source of those calories. You just have to eat what you can keep down. After that, if you're able to make choices, then you can start to focus on micronutrients."

The human body has shown great resilience in functioning with a very limited diet through dire and demanding circumstances. During the Irish potato famine, much of the country's population had to depend on what they could forage when their crops failed. This led them to subsist on plants such as stinging nettle, wild mustard, sorrel, and watercress for some time. Individuals who are forced to function on limited nutrients and calories tend to lose a lot of weight, but for a few weeks or months our bodies are able to adapt and persist with just about any food source.

The first thing I wanted when I finished my trail record hike was sleep—the second was a steak. I was constantly craving protein on the record hike, and that desire was strongest in the morning. I was weak and lethargic until I could get nuts, eggs, or a sausage biscuit in my system. Overnight my energy stores smoldered like a dying fire. Protein was the fuel I needed to start that fire back up again. Once it was going, I could throw almost anything on it to produce heat and energy.

When I mentioned my protein craving to Shawn, he reminded me of an interesting fact that I'd learned in middle school science class: Our muscles are constantly rebuilding themselves; the cells are continuously breaking down and replacing themselves. Within fifty to a hundred days the cellular makeup of a hiker's bulging calf will completely turn over and you will have an entirely new leg muscle. Shawn suggested that the demands of a record attempt would accelerate that process. Because we need protein to rebuild muscle, it makes sense that I was daydreaming about steak, and fried chicken, and North Carolina pulled pork barbecue with vinegar sauce.

I felt vindicated in my carnivorous cravings but I also wondered about my endurance friends who are vegans or vegetarians. I wondered whether this high demand for protein might put them at a disadvantage. But according to Shawn protein is protein.

"There shouldn't be any appreciable difference in processing animal protein versus plant protein as long as you are getting enough," he said. Shawn went on to suggest that different people will have varying responses to diets and that what works well for one athlete might not be best suited for another.

I have witnessed elite hikers and runners perform at the highest level while proselytizing for a variety of different diets. Some forsake simple sugars and stick to the caveman diet; others prefer all-plant-based nutrition. I know many folks who have crossed gluten or dairy off the menu, and I have a few friends who believe that foraged and hunted foods are superior to the rest.

To be clear, I am not trying to identify the healthiest diet; this isn't an objective look at the vitamins, minerals, and macronutrients on any food plan or a discourse on the environmental impact of specific food sources. Bookstores dedicate entire sections to those topics, and with good cause. What I am saying is that when it comes to long-distance performance, I have witnessed a variety of meal plans used effectively. I have also heard from many a thru hiker and runner that his or her diet is superior to the rest. But I think what that person means, or rather what that person should say, is that it is the best diet for that specific individual.

Shawn provided the science to support my theory that what works for one person might not be the best fit for another. He said that each individual has distinctive microbiomes that help break down and process the food that we eat. All those probiotics that they sell us at the health food stores and in our yogurt help the microbiomes do their job. But even with the help of a good probiotic, different people, with different microbiomes, will respond to different foods—differently. The flora and fauna in our gut are nearly as unique as our DNA and are directly connected to it. Genetic heritage, ethnicity, and gender are all factors in our microbial makeup.

The takeaway here is that when you are standing in front on the diet section at your local bookstore looking for the right nutrition plan, and you are overwhelmed by the variety of options before you, perhaps the best thing you can do is trust your gut.

The many different physical considerations that Shawn and I discussed made me wonder if there's an ideal body type and constitution for endurance. And if there is, what would it look like?

Andrew Thompson shared with unyielding confidence that his physique was best suited for distance records. "My body type is directly in line with setting an FKT on the AT. I'm big, rugged, and can take a beating. If anyone should have an overuse injury it should be me! Nothing about my makeup suggests that I have covered tens of thousands of miles. My body can take it."

Despite Andrew's certainty, I still wanted to confer with Shawn. "If you were to build the *ultimate* long-distance athlete, what would he or she look like?" I asked.

"The person would have legs like tree trunks with muscles composed of slow-twitch fibers, the cardiovascular system to match, and he or she would be slightly less built above the waist."

Andrew Thompson certainly had legs like a mighty oak, but I was more waiflike above the waist than he was. So I had him there! Strong legs and a diminutive upper body is a common physique for hikers and, on the trail, we jokingly refer to it as T-Rex syndrome.

I have always been a T-Rex; hiking just made it worse. I remember how self-conscious I was in high school when I developed calves instead of breasts. It took hiking to make me appreciate my body, my build, and my beauty. Plus, no one in his or her right mind messes with a T-Rex.

My awkward developmental years were exacerbated by the fact that I reached my adult height of seventy-two inches in eighth grade. It was inconvenient at school dances and when shopping for blue jeans, but as a tennis and basketball player I always believed that height was an advantage. I assumed the same would hold true on an

FKT. Shawn, however, suggested that there would be a tradeoff for a long stride. As with the expression that the bigger they are the harder they fall, on an FKT, the taller they are, the more mass they have to move down the trail. In other words, long legs equals more bone mass and a heavier frame.

Hikers and backpackers are constantly trying to limit their weight. Regardless of whether it is in your backpack or on your body, the heavier the load that you carry, the more difficult it is to make miles. But you don't want to start the hike looking emaciated. You need a few extra pounds and some extra energy reserves to expend along the way. It is best to start the endeavor with a svelte physique; not too heavy, not too light, but just right. The ideal way to start any endurance event is to look and feel healthy.

It was entertaining to go back and forth with Shawn trying to build the ultimate endurance athlete. I felt as if we had a children's block toy in which the head, legs, and core of a figure could be twisted and combined in different ways. I would consider a medley that paired Andrew Thompson's legs, my T-Rex upper body, and Scott Williamson's core and diet. Then I would twist one of the blocks and contemplate a different approach altogether. But even if I could build perfect endurance athletes and give them ideal diets given their constitutions something uncontrollable could end their chance at a record.

A year or two after setting the record on the AT, I was experiencing tightness and pain in my right leg that made it uncomfortable to hike and very difficult to run. An MRI revealed a golf-ball-size cyst that had lodged itself behind my kneecap and limited the range of motion for my tendons, ligaments, and particularly my IT band. It was manageable on the record, but two years later I couldn't walk around the neighborhood without discomfort. The lump wasn't genetic, it wasn't dangerous, but it did affect everything from my right foot to my lower back. The doctor said it needed to be surgically removed and that it would take six months of physical therapy before I could start running. That was a long, cranky six months.

Physical health is a gift and a privilege. It is important that we try to care for our health and protect it, but even so it can be taken from us at a moment's notice. A large cyst is a relatively small matter, but a tumor, or stroke, or car accident can take away the freedom of movement that we take for granted. The lesson here is simple: Don't take it for granted! When you are moving, whether at a leisurely pace or during intense activity, appreciate your body and enjoy its capabilities.

I might not always be physically able to hike upward of fifty miles a day, but I'll always be glad that I did.

I didn't contact someone like Shawn or pursue endurance research before I began my record attempt, because I wanted to listen to my body more than statistics and explore my boundaries without feeling like an experiment. I didn't want to be told what I could or couldn't do by someone who didn't know me all that well.

The irony of diving into the science of endurance *after* setting a trail record is that my technique would probably look different if I were to attempt an FKT tomorrow. When I talked with Shawn, I reveled in the aspects of my strategy that seemed to be spot on. But I regretted other decisions, such as sleeping more than I probably should have. And if I had it to do again, I think I would opt for starting in the late spring rather than in the heat of the summer.

Nonetheless, I'm still grateful that I didn't delve too deeply into the biomechanics and energetics of endurance before setting out on a record hike. The hypothesis behind my experiment was more personal than what could be postulated and studied in a lab, and my internal discoveries on the trail were more important than the physical results. Science can help us determine what is possible, but it takes a whole lot more than reason to deliver the evidence of endurance.

As I was winding down my discussion with Shawn, there was one more question weighing heavily on my mind—and I hesitated to ask it. If the answer was different from what I thought it was, I didn't want to know I was wrong. But I finally worked up my courage.

"What about gender?" I asked a bit haltingly. "Do you think men have an advantage over women?"

Shawn's answer was immediate and firm. "No. No, I don't think that at all. There are many, many hypotheses about why a woman's abilities would be equal to or perhaps even better than a man's in a long-distance endeavor."

You would think that I would have been most relieved to hear that endurance isn't responsible for impaired cardiac function, but in reality I breathed a bigger sigh of relief hearing Shawn dismiss the gender gap. So much of my motivation, so much of my positive self-talk and confidence, came from telling myself that women were equal at endurance if not uniquely equipped for it. I would have taken atrial fibrillation over the feeling of inferiority. It felt liberating to know that I wouldn't have to live with either one.

Once I heard that my sex was not a disadvantage, I quickly shifted to wanting to know if women might have the upper hand on long-distance pursuits. I started spouting off all the theories that ran through my head during the two-thousand-plus miles I spent convincing myself that I belonged.

"On my record, I kept telling myself that being a woman was a positive. I mean, relatively speaking we have smaller frames and less bone density so that means less weight to carry. But we also have a higher body *mass* index, which we usually hate because we end up carrying more fat than men do and have a muffin top above the waistline of our blue jeans. But on a record attempt, that extra layer of fat is an extra energy reserve that men don't have. And a smaller frame also means we'd require less calories and water, right?"

I paused for a split second to take a breath, then continued. "Plus, we give birth. We give *birth*, Shawn! Don't you think the evolutionary practice of carrying a baby for nine months and enduring labor pains would give us an advantage? Don't you?"

Shawn gave a contrastingly measured response. "There are a lot of small factors that come into play," he said. "What we find is that over time they all have a role and when we add them all up, we find that women are going to do very well at these types of endeavors."

"Then at what specific distance do you think women become competitive?" I asked. "Is it five hundred miles? A thousand? What?"

"It's hard to pinpoint an exact distance," he said. "There are always many individual exceptions, so let's talk about 'on average.' Men will do better at any type of strength and power activity because they have greater muscle mass and testosterone. When it comes to aerobic and cardiovascular activities, men typically perform better because their bodies carry more oxygen and they have higher VO2 max levels [the amount of oxygen an athlete can use, typically measured in body weight per minute]."

But as we go longer and longer distances, the ability of the heart to distribute oxygen becomes less of a factor. When we get to one thousand miles, VO2 max matters very little and the lactic threshold matters very little. The physiological differences are almost out the window. As I said earlier, humans were not born to run a marathon, let alone a hundred-mile race. And we certainly weren't born to attempt thousand-mile FKTs.

Extreme exercise is a new thing. Our genes have never undergone any evolutionary pressure to get good at those distances or to create real differences between men and women for that sort of activity. Most likely there's very little sex difference in these multiweek, maybe even multiday, events and beyond. Instead I think women's real advantage might be psychological."

It was a bit surprising to hear a physiologist say that the deciding factor in an extremely physical pursuit might in fact be mental. I asked him what he meant.

"Well, this is speculative," Shawn said, "but it involves the evolutionary and biological role of females to birth and take care of children. Women are caregivers so they tend to think less about their own discomfort than about what they are doing for others. There is something that goes along with the capacity for motherhood and childbearing that allows women to just deal with chronic discomfort and engage in less self-pity. Honestly, in these types of endurance events I think that might be the tipping point."

Shawn might have just simultaneously explained how I set the record and why I will never be able to do it again. When I was going after the FKT, I put my needs first for forty-six days. Brew understood that and supported it. In his words, I was allowed to be a diva.

Someone once asked if that made me feel selfish. I had to be selfish to set the record. On the other hand, it was a rare opportunity to fulfill my dreams, and I don't feel guilty for seizing it.

After the birth of my daughter, a part of me knew that I would never again be able to pursue an extended FKT with success, but I couldn't articulate why, until now. My transition to motherhood did not take a physical toll that would prevent me from setting a trail record, but emotionally I am no longer capable of putting my needs first for forty-six days. As Shawn suggested, I'm wired to be a caregiver. It's my turn to help my daughter discover her dreams.

Ultimately, the question of gender and endurance is important to me not because I need to beat the boys—although I'll admit I like doing it. The men who have come before and after me in these endurance pursuits have been and will always be some of my greatest friends and role models. But it bothers me that my efforts and the accomplishments of so many female athletes have been treated as a fluke or second-rate endeavor.

For the past five years, Brew and I have purchased the same Christmas gift for each other. We buy VIP tickets to the Southern Conference College Basketball Tournament in our hometown. It's simple and there's no wrapping involved. Then, during the second week of March, we watch about forty hours' worth of live basketball over the course of five days. We immerse ourselves in the tournament to the point where I can hear whistles and buzzers in my head, long after we have left the gym.

At the tournament, I am struck by the fact that the women's games have a quarter of the attendees, yet very often they are better match-ups. There is no dunking or high flying in the women's competition, but because the teams can't rely on their physicality to win, they rely instead on strategy and teamwork. When you compare men's and women's athletics, there is no difference in intensity, dedication, or drama. The primary contrast is in pay and prime time.

We live in a culture that promotes men's sports and places women on the cover of athletic magazines as swimsuit models. And it takes individuals like Serena Williams, who has defied sexism, racism, and ageism throughout her twenty-year professional career, to show us that women's athletics can be as captivating as the men's draw and that women deserve equal exposure and equal pay.

This matters to me because I am a woman, an athlete, and clearly a Serena Williams fan, but most of all it matters to me because sports are a microcosm of our culture. Being a business professional, scientist, or politician doesn't have anything to do with bench presses and wind sprints, but females are still underrepresented and underpaid.

It's a well-reported and often-ignored fact that in America, women earn 70 percent of what their male colleagues take home, and we struggle for equal representation in high-paid professional pursuits, boardrooms, and politics. In our country's 240-year history, we have never had a female president.

The main reason that I love sports is that they can bring together different groups of people and redefine what is possible. The fact that I became the first woman to set the overall record on the Appalachian Trail holds some significance in the world of FKTs, but more than that I hope that it demonstrates that the farther we go, the longer we play this thing out, the closer we will come to the tipping point.

CHAPTER NINE

A Woman Rewriting the Rules

"More than anything, this was an internal journey."

—Heather Anderson

I was the first woman to set the overall record on the AT, but I was not the last. I've spent less time with Heather Anderson than with most of my other FKT friends, and yet I felt more connected to her than to any of the guys. We both hiked the Appalachian Trail straight out of college and completed the Pacific Crest Trail soon thereafter. We both set trail records and shook up the fraternity of FKT athletes. And we both answer way more questions about carrying guns and trail safety than any of our male counterparts. With Heather, there is a sense of sisterhood.

In the world of long-distance hiking, the percentage of females has steadily increased, but the trail is still dominated by men. Besides that, many of the women I see out there are often in groups or walking with a partner. It is rare to come across a woman like Heather who has spent much of her time in the backcountry alone.

When she's not on the trail, Heather lives in Edmonds, Washington. I flew out for a visit and we immediately started making plans for our upcoming adventure. It was late spring, and Heather wanted to climb one of the high peaks around Seattle. We may share a lot of similarities, but mountaineering is not one of them. Heather knew that I was not a technical climber, so I figured she would dial it down a notch. She told me that we could do an easy ascent, and then in the same breath announced her plans to take me on a ten-mile mountaineering expedition up Mount St. Helens. This was the same Mount St. Helens that gained international attention when it erupted in the early eighties. It is an active volcano whose summit is still covered in snow and ice in early June, and making it to the top would require the use of crampons and an ice axe. That's sisterhood for you.

I watched with hesitation as Heather and her boyfriend, Adam, threw their mountaineering hardware into piles. I looked down at the sharp spikes of the crampons and the pointed tip on the ice axe and decided that one way or another they were going to kill me.

They made three piles: one for Adam, one for Heather, and one for me. I started adding my designated gear to a pack that already brimmed with synthetic layers, a lightweight tent, sleeping bag, foam pad, trail snacks, three liters of water, and an extra-large first-aid kit. At least we had everything we needed to be safe and stay comfortable on the mountain. It was a far cry from the paltry rations that Heather and I each carried on our first Appalachian Trail hikes.

When I started my thru hike on the AT at the age of twenty-one, I had an external frame pack filled with a cumbersome synthetic sleeping bag, a four-season tent, a minuscule first-aid kit, and a plethora of Pop-Tarts and Slim Jims. I wore discount sneakers for the entire hike, used an old ski pole as a hiking stick, and when I lost the pole after six hundred miles, I replaced it and covered the remaining three-fourths of the trail with a fluorescent yellow mop stick. Still, my packing list was far superior to Heather's forty-pound load.

When she struck out from Springer Mountain, Georgia, Heather toted three cotton T-shirts, but no rain jacket or sleeping bag. Her foodstuffs consisted of five pounds of rolled oats and several bags of rice—*not* the instant kind. And the boots she bought at REI were too stiff and restrictive for her feet, which soon became flat and swollen from long days on the trail.

When she reached North Carolina she decided to take matters—and her feet—into her own hands. She cringed and hobbled down Standing Indian Mountain to reach the next trail wayside where she could take her shoes off and assess the damage.

"I remember when I arrived at Carter Gap Shelter, the tips of my toes had been bothering me all day. I found a blister under my toenail and decided to pop it. All this fluid shot out. Then I discovered I had blisters under every single toenail. I popped them all. And eventually I lost all of the toenails except for one. My feet were destroyed."

She hiked several more days and reached the southern boundary of Great Smoky Mountains National Park. There she decided the tent she had carried for the first 150 miles was too bulky, so she chose to mail it home. A lot of hikers mail home cumbersome items and replace them with lightweight alternatives, but Heather never replaced her shelter. As she worked her way across the Smokies, she spent the nights on the hard wooden floorboards of trail lean-tos, shivering herself to sleep under a space blanket.

When Heather started the trail, she had five hundred dollars to her name, and she was determined to make it to Maine without using credit cards or going into debt. To accomplish her goal, she procured food and gear from "hiker boxes," which are essentially recycling bins set up at hiker hostels, full of unwanted, unused paraphernalia. "I also dug stuff out of the trash," she said. "I still went hungry, but it didn't matter. Nothing was going to stop me."

When she arrived at a small town situated on a large bend of the French Broad River, she took two days off and searched for odd jobs. After earning fifty dollars, she went to the local outfitter and picked out the cheapest sleeping bag she could find, then she crossed the street to the Dollar General and bought blindingly white geriatric sneakers with Velcro straps. She wore the mall walkers into Pennsylvania, where she found a brand-new pair of New Balances in the hiker box. Never mind that they were three sizes too big. In Vermont, she traded the Pennsylvania kicks for another pair that was only *one* size too big, and those were the shoes she summited Katahdin in.

Along the journey, Heather methodically switched out her heavier gear for lighter, discarded options and generous hand-me-downs from people she met along the way. As her pack weight dropped, her confidence grew. In Virginia, her daily mileage increased and she became more consistent. She learned that she could hike consecutive thirty-mile days. The higher mileage also helped her to stay on budget, because it meant that she could go farther between resupply points.

Since she never replaced her tent, most nights she slept in trail shelters. On more than one occasion, a lean-to was full or she couldn't make it there at all. Those nights she cowboy camped and slept under the stars.

"One night when I was cowboy camping, I got chased down the trail by a moose."

"What, in the dark?"

"Yeah, I was in Maine and I woke up in the middle of the night to the sounds of a moose grunting and thrashing around next to me. I didn't carry a headlamp because I couldn't afford it. I just had a keychain light that another hiker gave me. But I got up as fast as I could and tried to start hiking up Barren Mountain in the dark.

"While I was packing camp, I broke my glasses and lost a lens so I could only see out of one eye. And I can't see more than six inches in front of me without my glasses. When I finally got up to the flat rocks on the ridge I decided to camp there under the moonlight . . . but even when I lay down, I could still hear the clopping of hooves on the rocks below me."

For several minutes, I couldn't stop laughing, nor could I shake the vision of Heather scrambling up the vertical rock jungle gym known as Barren Mountain, half-blind, in the dark, with a keychain light and a moose in hot pursuit. Finally, I composed myself and asked, "So, when you got to the end of the trail, did you know that you were hooked?"

Heather looked at me earnestly and said, "I didn't know in Maine. I knew in Virginia. I was *absolutely* hooked. I knew I was going to hike the PCT when I finished the AT. 'This is it,' I thought. 'This is what I'm doing for the rest of my life.' I love the challenge, the adventure, the physicality and being outdoors. It was. . . . It is just the perfect thing for me."

Heather spent the next year and a half working seasonal jobs at Glacier National Park in Montana and Jackson, Wyoming. She took a trip to the East Coast in the spring of 2004 to attend an annual Appalachian Trail festival known as Trail Days. There she met a young man named Remy who was currently on his own pilgrimage to Maine. They started off as pen pals, then became romantically involved, and shortly thereafter, they were engaged. Heather was twenty-two; Remy was nineteen.

In 2005, they started their thru hike on the Pacific Crest Trail as a couple. The beginning of their engagement—and their hike—was idyllic. "We were young and everything was perfect." But they began to experience the usual partner conflicts. When you are hiking 2,663 miles with someone, there are *always* kinks to be worked out.

"At one point," she said, "I was so frustrated with him that I threw my pack down and shouted, 'I'm leaving!' When I started to walk away, he waited a second, then said, 'Um, aren't you going to need your pack?' So I stopped in my tracks, walked back toward him, picked up my pack, and continued hiking down the trail in the direction we'd been going."

It's hard to walk away from someone when you're hiking the same trail.

After working their way through the scorching temperatures and exposed terrain of the Southern California desert, Remy and Heather made it to the snow-capped peaks of the Sierra Nevada. By this point they had fallen in lock step with each other. Their arguments decreased as their daily mileage increased. But when they stopped near Forester Pass to draw water from a patch of snow, they met two men who were putting in longer days and greater distances than anyone they had come across.

Just two months after I first met David Horton running up The

Priest on the Appalachian Trail, Heather and Remy crossed paths with him on his PCT. But this time he wasn't alone; he was accompanied by his friend and competitor "Flyin' Brian" Robinson.

The first widely recognized, fastest known time on the PCT was established in 2001, when Flyin' Brian hiked the trail in eighty-four days. His West Coast record was part of a much larger accomplishment. That same year he hiked the Appalachian Trail and the thirty-one-hundred-mile Continental Divide Trail. The hikers who complete all three footpaths are considered Triple Crowners. They are hiking royalty. Most consider a Triple Crown to be a lifetime achievement; Flyin' Brian completed his in a calendar year. He established one FKT on three combined trails—and set a PCT record along the way.

In 2005, David Horton was trying to surpass Brian's mark on the PCT. The fact that he had a support crew and was simply attempting a 2,663-mile record versus an 8,000-mile record gave him an advantage. His other big advantage was Brian Robinson. In a show of camaraderie and selflessness, Brian came out to assist David on a long stretch of trail where there was no road access.

"When I met Horty and Brian, that's when I started thinking about trail records," Heather recalls. "Remy and I had another eighteen hundred miles on the Pacific Crest Trail to think about what Brian had accomplished and what David was doing."

When Heather reached Washington, she looked at Remy, then she looked down at her washboard abs and strong legs, then she looked back at her gaunt boyfriend and took note. She surmised that women might be well suited—or even *better* suited—for long-distance travel than men. "It just didn't seem to take the same physical toll on women. The ones I saw at the end of a long hike looked fit and badass; the guys looked emaciated."

As soon as the duo finished the Pacific Crest Trail, they made plans to hike the Continental Divide Trail the following year. By that point they were completely in sync. After completing the CDT, Heather and Remy were married.

Heather's boyfriend, Adam, drove as we made our way through Seattle's viscous traffic pattern and then down Interstate 5. Our short
car trip was filled with trail stories that made me feel that Heather
and I had fought different battles in the same war. I could visualize in
detail the scene of nearly every anecdote she delivered. The familiar-
ity deepened our laughter, prolonged the gasps, and negated the need
for much backstory.

When we exited the interstate and the roads were no longer
straight, I gazed toward the horizon and was struck with a sense of
wonder and freedom as I took in the distant mountains. On the East
Coast, our largest mountains are interconnected—more a single
spine than a series of peaks. But the volcanoes in Washington and
Oregon rise out of the valley floor like imposing, isolated giants.

I focused on the view while Adam and Heather discussed their
plans for the upcoming winter.

"We could spend a month or two in Guatemala, then go to Ecua-
dor," Heather offered.

"That could work," Adam said. "Then maybe we could spend a
week or two in Cuba on our way home."

"Or we could go to Indonesia and get some more climbing in,"
suggested Heather. "But if we travel that far I want to stay for at least
six months."

While my companions debated the merits of peak-bagging for
three months in Central and South America or spending half a year
climbing in Indonesia, a part of me wondered whether an uneasiness
in my stomach was due to the windy back roads or regret.

I had enjoyed more backpacking in a decade than most people enjoy in a lifetime. Even now Brew and I give each other two weeks a year
for solo hiking excursions. But I remember when all I did was work to
hike, when six months a year spent on the trail was acceptable—and
expected. I have given that up. And there are times—times like
these—when I miss it.

_____

When we pulled up to the campers' bivouac nestled in the forest, we found a reasonably flat spot, pitched our tents, and rolled out our well-worn gear on the silnylon floor, then ate our dinners cold, brushed out teeth, and retreated into our respective shelters.

The sun was setting. I was ready for bed, but instead of being serenaded to sleep by nature, I was kept awake by the car-camping Seattleites and Portlanders who were blowing up ten-inch-thick air mattresses, pounding heavy tent stakes into the ground, and laughing and drinking beer from the comfort of their camp chairs. It's a little bit of an oddity and somewhat pitiful to be a thru hiker amid a community of car campers.

With our muted, minimalist gear; the silent, efficient way we set up our tents; and the fact that no one in our group even mentioned a campfire, we blended into the background so much that the other campers didn't even know we were there. At this point in life, I love blending into the background, but there were times growing up when it was terribly lonely.

Beyond our common obsession with long-distance hiking, Heather and I both abhorred high school. I realize that a lot of young women hate high school. But too often it seems the struggles of adolescent girls—with bullying, eating disorders, anxiety, and sexual harassment—are portrayed by Hollywood as rites of passage rather than issues that need to be confronted, so talking through them in an authentic way with Heather felt like a communion of two souls.

Heather went to a local public school in Middleton, Michigan, where the same forty kids progressed together from kindergarten to twelfth grade. Heather had been on the low end of the pecking order at age five and it just got worse from there.

"I got picked on all the time," she recalled. "I was the smart kid and as I time went on, I also became overweight. I was made fun of, bullied, ostracized. I had a few friends at school but not many. There were times I didn't want to be around other people. I got used to spending time by myself and doing things by myself."

There was no way out of her K-12 education in Middleton, Michigan, so Heather had to find a way to get through it. She escaped into reading books, writing poetry, and exploring the twenty-eight-acre property that surrounded her home.

As she grew, her connection to nature became less recreational and more utilitarian. Her dad worked in an auto factory fifty miles away. When he came home she would help him gather wood and stack logs for the stove that heated their home. She worked beside her parents in the family garden and helped her mother in the kitchen when it was time to can vegetables. Hard work outdoors did not make her resentful of nature. If anything, it enhanced her connection with the environment.

Despite her chores, Heather did not consider herself athletic or outdoorsy in any way. As a youth, she had a strong, stocky build. The only time Heather was courted for a sports team was when the track coach thought she might make a decent shot and discus thrower. The same woman who is now a top finisher in fifty- and hundred-mile races was never asked to run because she didn't have the body for it. Twenty years later, Heather's physique resembles that of a strong, svelte Greek goddess, with calves so defined that they could cut diamonds. It is amazing the physique and physiology that can be uncovered by new experiences.

Heather internalized the negative comments of her peers and struggled with insecurity and self-image throughout high school. She found refuge in food, masking her negative emotions in the dopamine release of a sugar binge and hiding behind the pounds that accumulated on her five-foot-eight-inch frame. By the time she graduated, she weighed two hundred pounds.

She could hardly wait to leave Michigan and go to college somewhere—anywhere—else. Heather Anderson decided on Anderson University in Anderson, Indiana. "My mailing address was a little repetitive," she says, "but overall it was a good fit."

At college, she had friends in her classes and in her dorm. She was finally in an environment where being studious was valued and encouraged. But she also had access three times a day to an excess of food in the college cafeteria. As a result, she continued to put on weight.

Heather's freshman diet consisted of starving herself, then bingeing. She never sought professional help and confesses that she didn't fully heal from her unhealthy eating habits and the depression that followed for many years. Ironically, it was a summer spent at the biggest gorge in the country that set her on the right path.

After wrapping up her freshman year, Heather wanted two things: She wanted out of the Midwest and she wanted an adventure. So Heather took a job as a concessionaire at the Grand Canyon. "That was where I took my first hike," she said. "Even though I was overweight and out of shape, I could still hike."

The impact was life changing.

"It was the perfect combination of doing something challenging and beautiful," said Heather. "It was an adventure."

She hiked seventy-five miles that summer, a distance that at the time seemed incredible. One of the things that makes walking outdoors so special and appealing is that regardless of whether you travel a few hundred yards, a few miles, or fifty miles, you're a hiker. And now that Heather was a hiker she wanted to do more. Much more.

During her sophomore year, Heather made plans to hike the Appalachian Trail after college. Part of the process involved trying to lose weight and get in shape. One day she went to the track at Anderson University and started jogging. She made it halfway around and stopped. She couldn't jog any farther, so she walked the remaining two hundred yards to complete the lap. Then she started jogging again.

She couldn't go more than half a lap without needing to take a break, but for Heather this was much more than a two-hundred-yard shuffle. This was a building block toward being able to complete a full lap, then a full mile. This was a building block toward becoming a runner and a long-distance hiker. Those two hundred yards set a foundation that Heather would build her FKT dynasty upon. Endurance is not measured by someone's first steps; it is measured by her last step.

The following summer, Heather worked as a historical interpreter and tour guide at Mackinac Island State Park between the Upper and Lower peninsulas of Michigan. She spent the heat of the day in a full-length petticoat, long-sleeved dress, and hair bonnet cooking bubbling soups and savory stews over an open fire in eighteenth-century period garb. When she wasn't stationed in the kitchen, she was spinning wool, hand quilting, making soaps and candles, and demonstrating blacksmithing techniques. But before—and after—work, she tried to hike and run as much as possible. By the end of the season she managed to jog the entire perimeter of the island, a distance of eight miles.

She returned to school that fall and started running five to eight miles a day. She could now complete more than twenty laps around the same track where just a year before she had struggled to jog two hundred yards.

The following spring, after only three years, Heather completed her degree at Anderson University. She worked her way through school, received financial aid, and graduated early so that she wouldn't have to take out any student loans. She left without any debt—and she also left fifty pounds lighter than when she started.

My cell phone alarm sounded inside my tent at 1:30 a.m., and I heard Heather's go off a few seconds later. It was dark and quiet in the campground, but glimpses of brilliant stars through the evergreen canopy provided ample motivation to stay awake. We packed quickly, ate a breakfast of fruit and energy bars at the car, and started up the trail with our headlamps a little before 2:00 a.m.

Heather had suggested we wake up early to catch the sunrise from the rim of the volcano. The night before, it had sounded like a good idea—or at least one I was willing to go along with. But as we

ventured deeper and higher into the forest, mature fir trees blocked
out the stars. When the celestial light and directional bearings disappeared, I noticed that my headlamp was the dimmest in the group.
All I could make out was a small round orb of dirt trail and the occasional white avalanche lily lining the path.

Heather and Adam had both hiked this mountain before. They
knew where they were going. I felt content to follow the sound of their
voices and the distant glow of their headlamps bouncing up the trail.

When Heather worked as a historical interpreter at Mackinac Island,
she felt a special connection to her great-great-grandmother, who
had lived in the region and was a full-blooded Native American. She
was part of the Anishinaabe, a large group encompassing many tribes
on the border between Canada and the United States. When Heather
took a trail name on the AT, she chose Anishinaabe in honor of her
ancestor. To cut down on confusion because of pronunciation and
spelling, she quickly shortened it to Anish.

Heather's great-great-grandmother bore twelve children, her
great-grandmother had thirteen, and her father was one of sixteen.
Her lineage is composed of industrious women, women who were
known for working just as hard in the field as in the kitchen. Women
who kept their families fed and warm through the harsh Michigan
winters. Women with an impressive track record for childbearing.

When Heather and Remy completed the Continental Divide Trail
and got married, they agreed that they would always be hikers. But
they also thought they would work their love of the trail into a more
traditional lifestyle; they wanted to explore and continue having adventures, but they also wanted to share a home and have children.

They moved to Bellingham, Washington. Together they rented a
small but cozy apartment there and Heather set to work decorating
the new place. She got an office job to help support Remy in his pursuit of higher education at Western Washington University. Soon she

was hosting dinner parties for their neighbors, classmates, and co-workers. Each morning she dressed in appropriate business attire and went to her office, where she sat behind a computer for eight hours. After work, she would go for a run by herself, then clean up around the house and cook supper. Sometimes Remy was there; often he was still in class or studying. By all accounts, Anish had settled in and settled down. She found herself in the midst of a new life—one she found "colossally boring."

Thru hikers often transition into ultrarunning as a way to spend time on the trail without having to leave their families and careers for extended periods. Heather was no different. She became a weekend warrior, putting in her forty hours during the week, then hitting the trail with friends and competing in fifty-kilometer races on the weekends.

As the months passed, Heather continued to put more time into her training runs, and she started to enter longer races. In 2010, she ran a 50-miler. The following year she completed her first 100-mile event. The woman whose college highlights included hiking 75 miles over an entire summer and jogging 8 miles around Mackinac Island was now completing 100 miles at a time. For most people that would be more than enough adventure. Heather described it as a "Band-Aid."

Meanwhile Remy's academics were becoming his own feat of endurance, constantly demanding more time and effort. Long-distance hikers are not known for their moderation, and such intemperance can spill into other areas of their lives.

Between 2008 and 2011, Heather and Remy did not tackle any more long-distance trails. And after four years of not hiking together, they decided to divorce.

"I don't regret anything," Heather said. "It was very amicable. We made the best decisions along the way that we could. It just wasn't working anymore."

There was a question I wanted to ask but didn't know if I should.

"You don't have to answer this if you don't want to . . ." I paused for emphasis, letting it sink in before I continued.

"Do you think you broke up because of the trail?"

Heather looked out the passenger seat window and I wished I could have seen her expression.

"We both changed," she said. "For Remy, hiking was a part of who he was. But for me it was everything. I didn't find anything in society to keep me there. I didn't have something else. I was homesick." (It took me a minute to realize Heather was referring to the trail.)

"I was desperate to be hiking all the time. I didn't want to work for the next number of years while Remy was in grad school. I realized that I didn't want to have kids and a family. I didn't want to settle down. Those were things that I didn't actually *want*; they were just things I was expected to have."

Too many times people think that endurance is all about grinding it out on the path where life has set you down. It's not. It's not a skill that's developed when you mindlessly follow the person in front of you. It is an ability that's honed when you make personal decisions about how to move forward and live your life. Endurance isn't accepting the trail you're on, it's choosing it.

It was fairly shocking and life changing for a young woman whose family tree included forty-one births in three generations to realize that she did not want or need children. By the time she turned thirty, Heather knew she didn't have to follow in anyone else's footsteps.

After two miles of hiking past ancient fir trees and sidestepping thick, low-hanging branches in the forest, the trail up Mount St. Helens exited the tree line.

There they were again, those brilliant, bright stars, unadulterated by any sort of light pollution. I could see much better on the exposed slope, and the cool breeze was a welcome relief on my warm, damp skin. My breathing was more rhythmic and less shallow, but the hiking wasn't any easier. The trail meandered through a giant boulder field that required scrambling up and over the sharp, granular surface of large volcanic rocks. The coarse pumice cut into my fingers and palms and I bruised my shins over and over again when my leg failed to fully clear a hurdle. The boulder field made the route unclear, but with frozen snow chutes to our right and left, we knew the only option was to stay on the rocks and pull ourselves higher up the mountain.

When Heather and Remy divorced in 2011, she knew it was the right decision, but that didn't make it any easier. She was now free to hike, but she couldn't get past the feelings of failure, not just in marriage but in life. She said, "I wasn't good at being normal."

Not wanting to make any rash decisions, she kept her job and stayed in Washington for another year. In time she started dating again, but nothing stuck. The following summer she decided to take a break from work—and relationships—and hike the Pacific Crest Trail through Oregon and Washington.

"I got out there and it was a tough readjustment," she said. "I hadn't been long-distance hiking in five years, but once I worked through my emotional issues and started dealing with the trail issues like mosquitoes and snow, I thought, 'This is *great!*'"

She was home again with her first love. By the time she finished her hike at White Pass in Washington, she had decided she would go back to the Pacific Crest Trail the following spring and try for a record.

"I had nothing else in my life," she said. "I had pretty much moved on from everything. I just had a dream to do this, to thru-hike and find out how fast I could do it."

At that point in time, Scott Williamson had set the mark at sixty-four days. Almost everyone thought his record would be impossible to surpass. This was, after all, *Scott Williamson*, the fifty-five-thousand-mile long trail veteran, the only person who had completed a PCT yo-yo, and the man who had set the West Coast's FKT *three times.*

"I didn't think I could break it," Heather admitted. "But there wasn't a female record. I thought the trail could be hiked in two months. Sixty days was a nice round number and I figured if I set this goal and stayed close, then even when I fell off pace I could still set a women's record. I decided if nobody else was going to try it, then I would. I was very certain that I was going to fail."

The first few weeks were excruciating. Despite having a year to prepare, she arrived at the trail nursing a hurt knee and feeling undertrained. After three days, her knee injury was no longer a concern, because her entire body was in pain. She suffered through triple-digit heat, relentless wind, and waterless stretches of desert while maintaining a forty-one-mile-a-day average. The high temperatures and grueling physical demands made it hard to eat, and within the first ten days she lost ten pounds.

After two weeks on the trail she regained her appetite. But she still couldn't make it through the night—or rather the four or five hours she budgeted for rest—without being forced awake by muscle cramps. When they seized her body, Heather would grit her teeth and writhe in agony until the painful contraction released its grip. Then, she would fall back asleep—until the next contraction.

She had passed through the chaparral and the Joshua trees of the Mojave Desert and into the Tehachapi Mountains, but her jubilation at leaving Southern California behind was tempered by the fact that she was headed for the hardest part of the trail, the Sierra Nevada.

Most Pacific Crest Trail hikers consider the Sierras to be the most scenic—and rugged—section of the trail. Once you leave the range's southern end, you travel through remote wilderness and over snow-covered mountain passes for two hundred miles before crossing another road at Red's Meadow. Most hikers go over only one pass a day, because such a schedule allows you to avoid slick snow in the morning and half-melted slush in the late afternoon. Ideally, you want to reach the day's high point just after lunch, when the snow is soft, steady, and sounds like it is crunching beneath your shoes.

Heather knew that if she wanted to set the record she would have to cross not one but two passes each day, and that meant traversing ice-encrusted snowfields in the early morning hours. It also meant post-holing—or sinking up to her thighs in cold sludge throughout the late afternoon.

She checked off pass after pass, every ridgeline representing one fewer hurdle between her and Canada. But after climbing Forester, the highest point on the trail, she didn't know if she had the strength to make it over the next ridge. Glen Pass taunted her in the distance, seeming to move farther away with every step. As she climbed toward the jagged notch and felt her legs quivering beneath her, she placed the palms of her hands on her thighs to steady her gait and settle her mind. It suddenly felt as if she were breathing through a straw.

The trail was carved into the mountain, and a precipitous fall seemed as probable to her as making it up the pass. Feeling wobbly and weak, she pressed her flushed cheeks and throbbing temple against the cold granite and rested her weight against the sheer rock wall. She began to hyperventilate and feared attempting another step. So she stayed put. The seconds passed slowly because she was in so much pain, but the minutes passed quickly because every one counted. Eventually, her breath grew deeper and steadier, her legs felt stronger, and she took a step. She focused on taking one step, and then another, then another until she made the pass.

Looking out into the starlit sky, Heather could make out the black silhouettes of the mountains shrinking in the distance. She wasn't at the end of the trail, and she hadn't yet set a record, but the feeling Heather had at that moment made every step she had taken and every obstacle she had yet to overcome fully worthwhile.

The sense of pride that Heather felt after making it through the

Sierras left her feeling light and strong as she hiked through Northern California. But when she hit Oregon her energy reserves disappeared. She was depleted. This was supposed to be the least difficult part of the trail, a moving sidewalk compared to the mountain passes in the high Sierras, and yet it was proving difficult for her to lift one leg in front of the other.

"When I hit Diamond Peak Wilderness I started to fall apart," she said. "I had this weird ache in my triceps, my legs were giving out beneath me, and I was experiencing dizzy spells. I just started falling for no reason. My diet had been off since day one. I was anemic, and without knowing it, I was also gluten intolerant. I was consuming and absorbing very little protein. After two thousand miles, my body was at the stage of cannibalizing muscle tissue."

Heather stumbled into Big Lake Youth Camp to pick up her next resupply. She collected her package, then sat down to sort her food and repack her gear. But instead of being encouraged by her new provisions, she just started to weep.

"I sat there and I cried and cried. My body had had it. For several hours I sat there sobbing, feeling sorry for myself. I didn't think I could keep going. I didn't think I could set the record. But finally I told myself, 'Record or no record, you're going to finish this hike. You're still walking to Canada!'"

When she left Big Lake Youth Camp, she decided to add more protein to her diet, so at the next camp store she picked up as many tuna packets as she could carry. She was hesitant to carry this new staple through the heart of bear country, but as soon as she incorporated it into her meal plan, her body rebounded and her mileage increased.

Heather Anderson arrived at the Canadian border sixty days after leaving Mexico. She set the record; she took four full days off Scott Williamson's seemingly insurmountable time. She had told herself it was "reasonable" to hike the trail in sixty days, that if no one else was going to try it she would. She had thought she would probably fail. But she didn't.

She earned a little recognition, a lot of respect, and a long rest. On her record hike, she had told herself to hike through the pain, weakness, and extreme conditions. There was only one problem: Once it was over, she didn't know how to stop.

I needed to take a break and catch my breath before we reached the crater rim. The altitude was both humbling and abrupt. Heather and Adam, ever the gracious hosts and guides, rested as well. But every time I asked to take a break, I felt as if I were pulling on the reins of a runaway racehorse. When I needed to stop, I watched Heather create extra switchbacks in the rocks so that she could keep moving or chip at a nearby snow drift to see whether the top had iced over. At one break, she pulled a snack from her bag, not because she was hungry, but because eating gave her something to do. She kept glancing east, measuring our pace against the brightening horizon.

The sun rose before we reached the rim, but the view from the crest of the volcano was no less breathtaking. I felt accomplished and terrified. I was pleased with myself for hiking through the night to reach the crater rim, some eighty-three hundred feet above sea level. There I was, slightly panting and standing on the snow and ice that lined the volcano like salt on a margarita glass, staring into the gaping crater of an active volcano.

Despite the staggering beauty, there were signs of destruction everywhere. It was clear where the forest had been hit with lava flow, and steam vents rose from the valley floor. The landscape resembled the backdrop of Jurassic Park or a fourth grader's prehistoric diorama.

Suddenly we heard a reverberating crack, followed by an interminably long crashing sound coming from the crater's mouth. My body went rigid with fear. I was convinced that after thirty-six years, Mount St. Helens had timed its encore perfectly for our arrival.

"There it is," said Heather, pointing to the southern rim, as casually as if she had been showing me a can of beans that had fallen off a shelf in a grocery store.

"It's a rock fall," she said.

"Don't worry. It's normal," added Adam.

I looked at my friends in disbelief, then looked back at the plume of dust rising from the inner rim, where the last few rocks were colliding with the crater's basin. Heather and Adam's "normal" was not my normal.

We shared the rockslide and the sunrise with a group of four climbers. They, too, had hiked through the night to reach the rim. But as we pulled out our ice axes and debated whether to use microspikes or crampons, the other group turned around and headed back down the mountain. A part of me wanted to join them. Hadn't we accomplished what we set out to do?

"Most people who hike up here don't walk all the way to the summit," Heather explained.

"But the conditions are perfect today," chimed Adam. "The snow is soft but not slushy, and the slope isn't that steep. We shouldn't have any trouble making it to the top."

Heather, sensing my anxiety, added gently, "Jen, if you want you can wait here."

I looked out at the glistening white strip that stretched between us and the crown of the mountain. Then I gazed down at the serrated lava rocks where the snow cover had retreated. In my head, I repeated Adam's words, "The conditions are perfect. The snow is the right consistency and it's not even that steep."

"Can I hike between you two?" I asked.

I didn't trust myself, but I did have faith in my hiking partners, and they had confidence that I could make it to the summit.

"When I got to Canada, I couldn't process the record," Heather said. "A part of me wanted to forget that it happened. I had nightmares for months. In my dreams I was always hiking, I always had farther to go and there was something that kept me from getting there. At first, I dreamed that I was hiking down a path filled with venomous snakes. Later I dreamed that I just broke down—that I couldn't go any farther. It took me six or eight months to come to terms with what I had been through. But even then, I thought it was an accident. I thought, 'I'm not anything special so how did it happen?'"

After the record, Heather went home to another romantic relationship that soon ended and a job at a health food store that she didn't like. She spent much of her spare time entertaining hiking clubs and outdoor audiences with her story of setting the PCT record. She drove for hours and spent her own money on gas to tell people what it was like to hike forty-five miles per day.

But with every talk she felt more and more like a fake. It was easier for her to believe that some sort of cosmic coincidence had led to the record, rather than her own ability.

In the summer of 2014, the year after her PCT record, she went after the FKT on the 211-mile John Muir Trail, which is synonymous with the PCT through much of the Sierras.

"I failed miserably," Heather said.

"You just didn't acclimate," Adam interjected. "You needed more time." Adam and Heather started dating right before she left for the John Muir Trail. After it, Heather flew to Colorado to give another talk on her PCT record.

But, she says, "That was it. That was the last one. I couldn't do it anymore. I couldn't talk about the PCT. I deleted my presentation from my computer and refused to give talks. I realized that I'd left the trail physically but I never moved on emotionally, and it was time to create space."

In just sixty days, Heather had gone from being a young divorcee who loathed her job to a hiking celebrity with a mountain of expectations. Adam was right; she needed more time to acclimate.

When she returned from Colorado, she started actively pursuing mountaineering adventures in Washington State. She quickly became more comfortable with elevation, and whenever she could she began challenging herself on solo climbs, adventures with Adam, or outings with a group of friends.

Adam had begun peak-bagging before Heather, and he had tagged more summits. But she quickly caught up, both in her ability and in her tally.

Heather had been in multiple relationships with guys who tried to match her step for step. And she had also had boyfriends who stayed at home while she tackled adventure after adventure. But she had never found someone who could give her both companionship and independence until she met Adam.

I loved watching the two of them interact. On countless occasions, Adam reached out to grab Heather's hand or Heather walked into Adam to press herself against his side and nuzzle her forehead against his shoulder.

Heather and Adam still had energy for adventures and each other.

When I asked Heather questions, Adam often interjected to mitigate a self-deprecating answer. I appreciated his feedback. There are things a partner notices that a mirror won't detect.

I also loved hearing Adam's take because his affection for Heather came across as honest and endearingly awkward.

"I was fascinated by Heather before I even met her," said Adam.

"I heard about her from some mutual climbing friends and remember thinking, "Wow, what she is doing is so inspirational!" When we met, I realized we wanted the same things out of life. We were going the same direction."

Adam started hoping and believing that he and Heather shared enough—as he puts it—"common ground" to walk through life together. He fell in love with a woman who loves the trail and is committed to adventure and with a woman who did not want to be tied down to caring for a home or children, but he fell in love with much more than an idea or a road map for life. He fell in love with Heather.

"She's the most supportive, gentle spirit that I've ever met. I've never been so happy. I feel like a better person now that she's in my life.

❧

When Heather decided to go after the self-supported record on the Appalachian Trail in 2015, Adam believed that she would set it. "I just *knew* she would," he said. But Heather wasn't so sure.

"I've always had this feeling of inadequacy," she admitted. "Even after setting the PCT record, I still struggled with self-esteem and had trouble believing in myself. I knew the only way to put those voices to rest was to go back and do it again, this time on the AT. I wanted to hike to Springer Mountain—to go back to where it all started—because I needed to prove to myself that I had value and self-worth, that I was athletic and capable. More than anything, this was an internal journey."

Heather chose to pursue an externally demanding endeavor to mimic her inward quest. This time she had a better handle on her diet and she knew how to train properly. "It felt like the right time, the right place, and the right trail to really push my body."

The trail pushed back.

Heather was stopped not once but twice in the first two weeks at high river crossings in Maine and New Hampshire. Arriving in the evening without any viable options for fording the swollen channels, she opted for the most mentally challenging thing a person can do on a record attempt: She waited. Heather, an endurance athlete whose greatest strength was the ability to crush miles while sleep deprived, spent fifteen hours reclining on the banks of the Kennebec River, and nine more sleeping beside Cascade Brook.

Both times, she rested and wrestled with the fact that the downstream current seemed to be carrying away the record—and her self-worth.

Mountaineers have an adage that more or less says, It's one thing to get up a mountain, but it's another thing entirely to make it back down safely. It is a testament to Heather's maturity and adaptability that on a journey where the clock mattered so much, she chose to wait until the water levels dropped before pressing onward.

Because of the high water, Heather was off her schedule by the time she exited New Hampshire. It was demoralizing to be so far behind so early into her hike. So Heather opted to completely disregard her original itinerary. She decided to stop focusing on what other people had accomplished and, instead, concentrate on the simple task of putting one foot in front of the other.

In New England, she dealt with high rapids and heavy storms, but when she reached Pennsylvania the state was in a severe drought. Time after time she came to a water source that was listed in the guidebook as reliable only to find nothing more than some damp moss-covered rocks and a fetid mud puddle. Rather than worry about seasonal water sources and springs, Heather made the decision to carry more water—at times adding five pounds of liquid weight to her pack.

She carried her sloshing pack over the rock-strewn ridges of Pennsylvania, some of the most tedious, uncomfortable stretches of trail imaginable. She survived the scalding ridgelines of the Mid-Atlantic and continued to make good time through Virginia. She was now losing noticeable daylight in the morning and evening, but that didn't matter to Heather.

"I came alive at night," she said.

And so did the forest. "I heard and saw so many more animals in the dark."

Late one night she found herself alone on a ridge when suddenly she heard an animal ahead of her. Squinting, she couldn't quite make out its shape, but she clearly saw the glow of its eyes reflected in her headlamp. Everything about the encounter, the creature's furtive movements, its approximate height and size, and its intense scrutiny of her approach, told her she was staring at a mountain lion. But this wasn't California, this was a forested ridge surrounded by rural Virginia farmland along Interstate 81. She doubted her initial assessment and determined it must be a bear or wild boar. At some point, she decided it didn't matter; whatever it was, she was getting closer to it and she wasn't going to let it intimidate her.

"Get out of my way!" she screamed.

The animal ran off. Anishinaabe didn't even break stride.

By the time she reached North Carolina, Heather was on pace to break the self-supported record established by Matt Kirk in 2013. Matt, a lanky wisp of an endurance athlete, had won 100-milers and set numerous trail records in the Southeast. He also happened to be the first person to move the self-supported mark on the Appalachian Trail to under sixty days. In so doing, he broke the record Ward Leonard established back in 1990. It had taken more than twenty years to take twenty-four hours off the self-supported record. When Heather exited the Smoky Mountains, she found herself on pace to lower it by four days.

The only time she slowed down was when she reached Wayah Bald and found a group of students from a nearby university who were banding migratory birds. The birds would unwittingly fly into thin netting the researchers had stretched between nearby trees. They were then collected and given temporary housing in brown paper lunch bags to allow time for the students to record information and clasp a small metal band around the bird's leg. At the end of this process, a student would lift the paper bag holding the bird toward the sky and the bird would fly off unharmed.

Heather was walking past the group with a curious look on her face when the teacher noticed her.

"Hi," he said. "Are you thru hiking?"

Heather nodded.

"Would you like to release a bird?"

"That would be awesome!" Heather said.

He walked toward her holding one of his birds. She held out her hands and carefully received the small bird poking its head out of the crinkled bag. It looked fragile and frightened, but when Heather gripped it she could feel the strength of its wings and the warmth of it breast through its paper-thin housing.

"Time to let her go back into the wild," prompted the instructor, smiling.

Heather loosened her grip and raised her hands to the sky. The bird paused momentarily, then launched itself away from its paper bag and into the air. Heather watched until it flew out of sight. Then she kept hiking.

Despite my fear of walking that last quarter mile between the crest of the crater's rim and top of Mount St. Helens, I was pleased with how quickly and easily the traverse went by. I was surprised when Adam announced that we had reached the summit. I looked up from my boots, which I had been fixated on for the past thousand or so feet, and found that we truly were at the highest point

We had hiked through the suffocating darkness of the forest and scrambled over shards of igneous rock by the light of the moon. Despite my inexperience with crampons, ice axes, and all things alpine, there I was on top of a mountain with climbers and close friends who never doubted I would make it.

Now all we had to do was hike back down the mountain. But before we descended, Heather turned to me and asked, "Hey you don't happen to have a tampon, do you?" I dug in my pack and handed her one.

That may sound ordinary or inappropriate depending on how comfortable you are with menstruation, but for me it was a moment. There we were, seemingly on top of the world, exhibiting our strength, sharing our vulnerability, and leaning into our womanhood.

Twelve years after first setting foot on the Appalachian Trail as an unprepared college graduate, and fifty-four days after leaving Katahdin on her record attempt, Heather reached Springer Mountain, claiming her second self-supported FKT and at the same time dethroning another demigod in the world of endurance hiking. She became the first person to hold a record on the AT and the PCT at the same time.

Most people thought Matt Kirk and Scott Williamson had the résumés, the makeup, the genetic composition, and the knowledge to put the Appalachian Trail and Pacific Crest Trail records out of reach. And they did. Then Heather Anderson came along, and she didn't just eke out a new mark; she eclipsed the records by more than half a week.

I proved that women could compete with the men. But Heather took it a step further and made everyone wonder if women were better than men at endurance endeavors. She not only redefines what is popular within a sport, she offers a new definition of femininity. She does not find contentment and fulfillment in a husband or children, but feeds her soul by searching for her physical limits in the wilderness.

This wasn't about besting other hikers or surpassing marks set by men. It was an internal journey and it had an intrinsic reward. "I came away from the Appalachian Trail a more confident and healthy person," said Heather. "My insecurities were put to bed. When I reached the end, I felt free."

Within a few days of setting the record, Heather was back in Washington and headed out to the Cascades with Adam for a multiday expedition. This time she had figured out how to let go of the past and move with confidence into her next endeavor.

On our drive back to Heather and Adam's, my feet were throbbing, my muscles were sore, every part of me ached with exhaustion.

Heather was in incredible shape. She could easily have turned around and hiked back up Mount St. Helens, treating the volcano like a casual workout of hill repeats. I was inspired by her conditioning and impressed with her drive to push herself.

But I wasn't jealous.

Someday I would love to climb volcanoes in Guatemala or spend six months exploring Indonesia. But during this season of my life, there is nowhere I'd rather be than with my family. Maybe what Heather and I have most in common is that we made conscious decisions—arguably more so than our male counterparts—about whether we wanted to give our time and energy to family or to the trail.

Through her conscious choices and deliberate actions, Heather has demonstrated that women can spend extended time in the wilderness and pursue extreme athletics while finding contentment—and femininity—in adventure. She has a family in the trail community, she has a home in the mountains, and she has two of the most dominant FKTs ever recorded.

CHAPTER TEN

The Genuine Celebrity

"I became not only empowered as an athlete but as an individual."

Scott Jurek

S cott Jurek is an anomaly in the ultrarunning and fastest-known-time community. Amid a small population of endurance athletes—the introverts, overachievers, and eccentrics who escape society by going as far as they possibly can into the woods—Scott Jurek has become a mainstream icon.

He has a social media following of several hundred thousand fans, and he was the star of the international best-selling book *Born to Run*. In 2014, he penned his own *New York Times* best seller. Scott travels the country giving talks and making appearances to promote his sponsors and share his message of active living and nutrition.

I had read the articles, books, and posts and felt as if I had a strong sense of the man behind each narrative. Yet after visiting with him, I had more follow-up questions about his life and his record than I did with any other record setter. The information I had didn't get me any closer to Scott and, in a way, presented a barrier. It is not difficult to learn about Scott Jurek; it is challenging to get to know him.

I reached out to Scott in March to see if I could set up a hike and conversation with him the following August. He immediately agreed to meet with me. But then it took a few months to nail down a possible window, after that it was difficult to lock down a day, and then there was a chance he would have to cancel our meeting because his sponsors had work for him in France. I had resigned myself to postponing and, I hoped, rescheduling, but then Europe fell through and we were back on. Maybe. On top of his full travel, work, and training schedule, he and his wife, Jenny, had welcomed a daughter into the world that spring and they were both busy caring for a newborn.

As our tentative meeting date drew near, I had more and more reason to doubt that our rendezvous would materialize. I boarded a plane and flew to Colorado on faith. My meet up with Scott still wasn't finalized and even if we were able to connect, I knew that I wouldn't get much time with him. But I wasn't going to get any time with him by staying at home.

When I touched down in Denver, I received a text from Scott saying he could meet for a few hours at a coffee shop in Boulder the following morning.

I arrived at the coffee shop twenty minutes early. I wanted to be ready and waiting in order to maximize our time together. When Scott walked in, he was cradling his three-month-old daughter against his chest in a baby carrier. I gave Scott a side hug and snuck a peek at the baby, Raven, sleeping soundly against his chest.

Scott is a tall, fair-skinned Minnesota Viking. His wife, Jenny, is petite and approachable, with Eastern ancestry. Their daughter reaped the best of their combined genetic traits. Her skin was a soft glowing bronze, and her jet-black hair was as soft and fluffy as goose down. Scott shot me a smile and stroked his open palms up and down on the outside of the baby carrier. Before I asked him any questions that morning, it was already clear what Scott was most proud of in life. He wore fatherhood well.

Scott's relationship with his own father was something he struggled with for most of his childhood and into his young adult life. Scott loved his father, but he needed more from him than his dad was able to provide.

Gordon Jurek was as imposing as the winter that howled outside their rural house in Proctor, Minnesota. The man was as cold as the subzero temperatures, as fierce as the biting wind, and yet interwoven throughout the harsh conditions there was undeniable strength and strange appeal.

Gordon worked extremely hard and at times held down two jobs to support the family. He went to a factory each morning to operate the boiler system during the day, then at night he moonlighted as maintenance staff at the nearby hospital. When Scott's dad was at home, there was work to be done around the house. The garden needed attention, the wood was waiting to be cut and stacked, and it seemed that if Scott and his two younger siblings weren't helping, then they were in the way.

"Sometimes you just do things." That was the motto his dad lived by, said Scott.

From sunup to sundown and well into the night, Gordon was a doer. He worked constantly to try to meet the bare minimum of what was required to live and to raise a family. Even with a job and a working garden, Scott's family still used food stamps at the grocery store.

Yet, as a child, what Scott needed from his father was not more money; it never bothered him that his family didn't use cash in the checkout line. He didn't mind spending his afternoons pruning the vegetables, starting the wood stove, or cooking for his siblings; he enjoyed working around the house. What Scott needed from his father was more time and affection. That would have helped a lot, but it still could not have met his deepest want. Because what Scott wanted most was his mother.

Scott remembers his mother when she was well. That makes it harder.

Up until the time he started kindergarten, Scott's mom played with him and read to him out loud, helped him learn to do things around the house, and taught him how to cook. Even though Scott had a sister who was born three years after he was and a little brother who was born two years after that, there always seemed to be more than enough love, attention, and delicious food in his house for all three children.

Scott's mom, Lynn, was an amazing cook. For work, she traveled around northern Minnesota to provide cooking demonstrations, and she was regularly featured on the cable channel preparing some of her personal recipes. At home, Scott remembers standing next to his mother in the kitchen helping chop vegetables from the garden or cleaning a walleye fish that Scott's dad had caught at a nearby lake.

In the fall, Scott would pick apples from low-hanging branches and off the ground and his mother would transform them into bubbly, golden-brown pies that filled the house with the scent of cinnamon and cloves. Each season brought different ingredients, new recipes, and savory memories wafting through the house. Then the scents started to fade.

Scott noticed that his mother started to drop more utensils in the kitchen and her chopping wasn't as quick or confident as it had been in the past. He saw her get tired early in the day and not have the energy to play, or read, or cook.

When he was six years old his mother was diagnosed with multiple sclerosis. She stopped working, scaled back her cooking, and needed help getting around the house. With his father picking up extra work, Scott now helped his mother and took care of his two younger siblings.

"She had a very progressive form of MS. It wasn't responsive to treatment," said Scott. "I remember when my mother had full health, but it was such a small part of my life. I knew my mother more as sitting in a wheelchair, undergoing tests, and trying new drug therapies."

Scott paused and looked down at his daughter who started to stir against his chest. "Losing a mother definitely shaped me."

By the time he was in high school, Scott's mom could no longer walk without assistance. Gordon pulled his wife on a sled into the forest to watch their eldest son compete on the local high school's cross-country ski team.

Scott started cross-country skiing by default. His parents couldn't drive him to baseball practice or afford the team gear and uniform that football entailed. So Scott made the most of the long northern Minnesota winters and the forest tracks outside his front door to learn how to glide effortlessly on two narrow skis through the snow.

Fate worked in his favor. One glance at Scott's tall, lean build and it is clear that he was much better suited for cross-country skiing than for varsity football. He was a natural at the sport and he kept improving. As an upperclassman, he consistently finished toward the front of the pack. He wanted his mother to see him ski well. He wanted to make her proud.

Scott didn't want to add any more stress to an increasingly stressful, and ever declining, situation at home. It seemed the less competent his mother became, the more distant his father grew. Scott compensated, perhaps overcompensated, by being perfect.

Scott Jurek was valedictorian of his senior class. In his graduation address, he encouraged his fellow classmates to be different, help others, and try to achieve things—especially while they were still young. Scott tried hard to follow his own advice. He was good at helping others and achieving things, but as a straitlaced teenager, he struggled to find what made him stand out from a crowd. What made Scott Jurek, Scott Jurek?

"I had lived not just inches but yards within the lines etched by parents and teachers, bosses and coaches," said Scott.

For college, he stayed near home in order to be close to his family. He enrolled in Saint Scholastica and decided to major in physical therapy, so that when he graduated he could help other people— people like his mother. Scott earned high grades while working thirty hours a week to pay for his classes. He ran on the school's cross-country team, but it was still just a means to get in shape for winter ski season. "I wasn't passionate about it and I usually finished mid-pack," Scott said.

He was meeting and exceeding societal expectations, but more and more Scott was attracted to friends and mentors who were punks and hippies, individuals who seemingly lived on the fringe. Maybe Scott could discover what made him different if he grew out his hair or started acquiring tattoos? Maybe if he lived out of his van for a while he wouldn't feel as grounded by convention? But Scott was not a rebel or a hippie. The fact is that Scott Jurek was a dork.

Then, midway through his master's degree, the cross-training for skiing became more enticing than strapping blades on his feet and gliding in straight lines. Running, especially long-distance running, felt dynamic. He could quickly change directions and spontaneously decide to explore different routes. He wasn't as limited by the terrain or landscape. His feet could take him places that his skis could not. And, if he wanted to, he could travel as far.

Long-distance running appealed to Scott's transient soul and his conventional roots. He could be studious and disciplined during the week, but running through the starlit forest on freshly fallen snow and challenging his body to go farther and faster than it had before was his rebellion. Endurance running made Scott feel special. And, with time, it would make him special.

Scott ran his first marathon in 1994 and finished in a time of 2.54. But the race didn't seem long enough. For Scott, it was a first step. For his next race, he registered for the Minnesota Voyageur 50 Mile Trail Ultramarathon.

"The Voyageur 50-miler was the hardest thing I had ever done athletically," said Scott. He loved it. And he finished second.

"I started to think maybe I am okay at this," he said.

He graduated from his physical therapy program and started work, but in his spare time he was still very much still a student, except that now he was studying the philosophy, psychology, and physiology of endurance. Renowned physiologist Shawn Bearden has a research institute and graduate assistants at Idaho State to help him study physical performance. Scott Jurek had a PT office, library books, and his own body. They are both experts in their field.

As a lifelong athlete, Scott knew when he was at the maximum level of expenditure. He had met with the thunder and lightning of that euphoric and excruciating threshold on multiple occasions. He knew he wouldn't be successful by trying to run harder; instead he wanted to know how to run better.

Scott tweaked his diet. He started to focus on organic whole foods and vegetarian fare. He eventually transitioned to a vegan diet and at one point—like Scott Williamson—he consumed only raw foods. Scott Jurek ultimately brought cooking back into the fold because, in his words, "I spent too much time chewing on a raw foods diet." As he fine-tuned his diet, his performance increased, his race time decreased, and he started to recover faster between runs.

As a prolific reader, Scott collected a library of books covering the discipline and psychology of different athletes. He respectfully referred to these individuals as "existentialists in shorts." With each new book, he considered a new mind-set and gleaned at least one beneficial habit.

Scott started looking more broadly at philosophy and discovered Maslow's theory of self-actualization, a cerebral playbook for becoming the best version of your truest self. He identified with the concept of needing to fulfill basic needs before being able to maximize one's potential. So he worked hard to lay the proper physical and emotional foundations.

Scott also internalized Eastern teachings such as Bushido, or the samurai code. This ideology honors principles such as sincerity, bravery, honor, and self-control, but the samurai believed that the best state of mind was an empty state, in which the past and future were not distracting from the present moment.

As a runner, especially a distance runner, Scott needed to be in and of the moment. The past was exhausting and the future was daunting, but that single moment—a single footstep, then another—was simple. It was sacred.

Working as a physical therapist, Scott examined the body for

forty hours a week. His job was to observe injuries and foster reha-
bilitation. He became accustomed to watching the human physique
break down, and he became adept at helping it to heal. Scott had
daily access to exercise machines, medical devices, and research
technology that few other runners used. In between helping his cli-
ents, he turned his body into a laboratory. He carefully charted his
performance and measured recovery with factors such as VO2 and
heart rate and blood test results.

By equipping his mind with personal research, trends, and information, Scott learned how to run smarter, but he never let science
replace intuition or dictate his choices. He knew that performance
had more to do with the figurative heart than with physiology. Scott
approached his sport with sound logic and unbridled passion. And
his holistic methodology resulted in win, after win, after win.

More striking than the sheer number of Scott's victories is the quality
and diversity of his accomplishments.

He didn't just descend on Squaw Valley, California, and win the
most illustrious hundred mile race in the country. He claimed the
Western States Endurance Run title *seven* times in a row.

In 2005, two weeks after claiming his seventh victory on the trails
of the Sierra Nevada Mountains, Scott ran on the blistering roads of
Death Valley through 120-degree heat to finish first in the notorious
135-mile Badwater Ultramarathon and establish the course record.

Then, fifteen years after David Horton's Hardrock 100-miler
victory, Scott conquered that ultramarathon as well. It is one of the
most technical high-elevation races in the world, but the thirteen-
thousand-foot passes of Colorado's San Juan Mountains did not stop
the flatlander from Minnesota from, once again, setting the course
record.

Scott's adventures and accolades extended well beyond the bor-
ders of the United States. He traveled to the remote canyons of

northwest Mexico to prove his ability amid the legendary runners of the Tarahumara tribe. He flew to Greece and claimed a Spartathlon title by running 153 miles between Sparta and Athens faster than his competition. He then returned to Athens twice more to success-fully defend his title. And, in 2010, Scott ran for twenty-four hours around a 1-mile loop in Brive-la-Gaillarde, France, to set a new re-cord for the greatest distance completed in a single day by an Ameri-can, 165.7 miles.

Scott seemed to win, if not entirely control, nearly every race he en-tered. With so much success, no one ever thought that Scott Jurek might simultaneously be struggling with everything that he was losing. But his life was not nearly as perfect—or predictable—as his race results.

Once Scott was out of the house, his parents divorced, and at the premature age of forty-four, his mother entered a nursing home. She continued to lose motor function, and the television became her main source of companionship. As long as she could operate a remote, she felt that she had some independence and purpose, but eventually her fingers stopped responding, and she lost the ability to push buttons. She was trapped within her body, in a nursing home, watching TV shows that she did not want to watch but unable to switch channels.

Scott moved to Seattle in his midtwenties. The hardest part of living in the Pacific Northwest was not the rain; it was the distance from his mother. But the man knows how to work through distance even when it feels excruciating. He accepted that there was very little he could do for his mother back in Minnesota. It would only add to her pain to have Scott stay in the Proctor home and sacrifice his dreams in order to take care of her.

Scott tried as hard as he could to love his mother by living well. There was an inverse correlation between his mother's incremental loss of physical ability and Scott's rise to preeminence and optimized performance within the sport of ultrarunning. He vowed to never take his body or his ability for granted.

Scott spent his own funds and maxed out credit cards in order to arrive at the starting line of races throughout the country. He also refused to compromise his diet, and no matter how tight money was, Scott always opted for the best organic, plant-based fuel he could find. Purchasing the highest-quality food and plane tickets whose cost totaled more than the winner's purse was expensive. This fact, combined with lingering student loans and the expense of starting a physical therapy practice, left Scott struggling to get out of debt. Even as he started to obtain sponsors, the first fruits of those relationships came in the form of product, not payments or brand placement. And you can't eat running shoes—especially if you're a vegan.

By 2008, Scott Jurek was arguably the most accomplished ultra-runner in North American history. But he was still working hard as a physical therapist and private coach, and very few outside of the infinitesimal, yet impassioned, distance-running community knew who he was.

Then in 2009, *Born to Run* was published. It pitted the epic running ability and anthropological habits of the Tarahumara people, an indigenous tribe living a relatively untouched existence in Mexico's remote Copper Canyon, against the greatest ultrarunner of all time, Scott Jurek. The book became pop-culture enough to headline a *60 Minutes* episode.

Yet at the height of *Born to Run*'s popularity, Scott wasn't just losing a mother, he was also letting go of a twelve-year marriage to his wife, he was struggling through a strained relationship with a close friend who served as his crew chief and lead pacer at races, and monetarily he wasn't any better off. As he put it, "More notoriety doesn't always yield financial benefits."

The fact that Scott was thrust into the public eye didn't make him happier or wealthier—it just meant that everyone got to watch his life unravel. And this is where Scott differs from all the other FKT athletes. The rest of us live out our endurance in the woods and enjoy a normal existence at home. We can keep a low profile and hit the trail without being asked to stop every few hundred yards for a selfie. Scott Jurek lives his life exposed.

Scott runs and loves and loses in front of a crowd. And because of that, he can teach us something that no other record setter can. He can teach us how to pursue endurance when all eyes are on you. *Lesson number one: When everyone is watching, you'd better be on the right path—for you.*

For Scott, the commercial success of *Born to Run* was infused with confusion and personal loss. Scott realized that public perception would never be able to replace personal drive, and meeting other people's expectations didn't make him feel fulfilled. He started to question his relationships, his accomplishments, and his running. He grappled with whether the commitment to his passion and the people in his life had been worthwhile. He wondered if his effort to help others run farther and eat better was making a difference. Was he actually inspiring people? Did he still feel inspired?

Scott didn't have the answers and he couldn't seem to find them on the trail, so he asked a shaman in Seattle what she thought.

"You're a leader," she said. "You're a teacher. You have to keep doing that." Then she added, "You want to do this long walk; why haven't you done it?"

Scott left feeling somewhat validated, but also wishing the shaman had been more specific. He still questioned what type of leader he should be, and he wondered what his most important message was. He knew that he wanted to help people run farther and eat better and live more thoughtful lives. But Scott wasn't sure if he needed to pick a focus; he hoped he could do it all. And what did the shaman mean by a long walk? Didn't she know that Scott was a runner!?

Scott kept up his endorsement schedule and book events, and he continued to run races. He couldn't be confident of his impact as a leader, or teacher, but he knew that it was part of his nature to try to inspire people.

He also proactively worked to rediscover his love for running and adventure. He went to places such as Yosemite Valley to relearn the simplicity of putting one foot in front of the other, not by racing or even jogging, but by suspending a line between two trees and slack-lining. Popular at college campuses, slacklining is the act—or art—of balancing between two points while suspended in the air on a narrow strip of webbing. It was true Bushido. Living completely in the moment with an empty mind, focusing on one footstep, and another, until . . .

"Shit!" A fall. Followed by laughter. Then starting once again.

After his visit to Yosemite, Scott traveled to the imposing chasm where Heather Anderson first discovered that she was a hiker. Scott went to the Grand Canyon to hide in the long shadows of vertical rock and sip from the depth of the valley's inspiration. He ran a ninety-mile course through a remote portion of the national park, with a friend and without support. They were entirely self-sufficient in the endeavor, and they almost quit—they probably should have quit given the conditions and their lack of provisions. Two-thirds of the way through the journey, the outlook was dire. They were out of food, without the proper gear, and surrounded by unforgiving terrain, but despite the harshness of their circumstances they decided to keep going and, be it by years of accumulated skill or by dumb luck, they survived. Sometimes it takes surviving to make you feel alive.

But the biggest change, the most pleasant discovery for a man trying to rediscover himself, was a woman.

It would be hard not to feel taken with Jenny Uehisa. When I first met Jenny, she immediately drew me in with her laughter and captivated me with her effervescent personality. I appreciated how she demonstrated her intelligence through thoughtful inquisition. Later on, I learned from an incidental misstep that she is loyal and doesn't back down from a fight. And, along with that, I discovered her ability to forgive. When you add in her adventurous spirit and athletic life-style, it's easy to see why so many people adore Jenny, most of all Scott.

At first, they were just friends. They participated in the same running groups and they were both involved in the outdoor industry in Seattle.

"I was never interested in him back then," she said. In fact, it was Jenny who informed me that Scott was—and still is—a dork. "He, like, wore cutoff blue jeans and had his hair in a ponytail. I just never thought of him as boyfriend material."

The more I got to know Jenny, the more I got to know Scott. At the point where I couldn't seem to get past the media portrayal and repetitive answers to repetitive questions that had been posed to Scott countless times throughout the years, I turned to Jenny to get to know the real Scott. She helped him transition from a running celebrity back into a human being.

After Scott went through his divorce, Jenny did what any good friend would do: She tried to set him up with her single friends. Scott agreed to go out to dinner with a couple of her girlfriends. It gave him a good excuse to stay in touch with Jenny and give her an update on how things were going.

"It wasn't until he came to visit me at my new job in California that I saw a different side of Scott," Jenny said. "I told him to come visit me so I could set him up with one of my coworkers, but after spending a few days together I saw how nurturing he could be. He was so kind. He loved cooking and wanted to make meals for me. He didn't mind doing chores around the house. He really delights in taking care of other people. Suddenly, I didn't want to set him up with my friends anymore."

The hurt and the loss that Scott had suffered through ultimately made room for a new relationship. It was Jenny who helped Scott say good-bye to his mother when she finally passed, it was Jenny who gave up a great job in California to move to Boulder with Scott and start a life together, and it was Jenny who helped Scott begin the long walk foretold by the shaman.

After they were wed, Jenny and Scott decided that they would section hike the Pacific Crest Trail together. Scott had already experienced a large portion of the trail, when he helped crew David Horton through Washington State on his PCT record. Helping David made Scott want to experience the entire route—it also piqued his interest in FKTs. But he knew that he wanted to backpack the Pacific Crest Trail.

Jenny, a native West Coaster, shared an interest in backpacking the trail. The longing was there, even before the path's popularity spike caused by Cheryl Strayed's best-selling book, *Wild*.

Scott and Jenny decided the western footpath was a long walk they could share. So they set out and hiked 120 miles together. The next summer they picked up where they had left off and backpacked another 100 miles. For two ultrarunners, their mileage was so . . . so . . . reasonable.

"People don't realize that Jenny and I love strapping on packs and hiking," said Scott.

Jenny laughed, "We are probably going to set the slowest known time on that trail."

It was on the PCT where Scott first pitched the idea of going to the Appalachian Trail and trying to set a record. When Scott helped David Horton with his FKT out West, the isolation, the unknown, and most of all the distance of a long trail appealed to him. At the time, however, his race schedule was too intense to allow him to take the time needed to thru hike or try for a fastest known time.

Now things were different. Scott and Jenny were entering a new season of life. Scott wasn't competitively racing the way he had in the past, and he and Jenny both wanted to try to start a family. They were a team, and they were looking for new adventures. *Lesson number two: You can't always get faster, but you can always go farther.*

On May 27, 2016, I received a voicemail message from Scott. He let me know that he was at Springer Mountain, Georgia, and he was going to try to surpass my record on the Appalachian Trail.

I was surprised and a little anxious that an athlete as decorated as Scott Jurek was trying to set the FKT on the Appalachian Trail. My initial reaction was, "I hope he doesn't blow it—blow me—out of the water!"

But ultimately, it was Scott and Jenny who were in for the bigger surprise. The trail, the record, the experience was not what they anticipated. Scott had only been on thirty miles of the Appalachian Trail before starting his record attempt, and Jenny had never crewed him for more than twenty-four hours.

"We just did this on a whim," said Scott. "Had Jenny really known what we were getting into, she might not have signed up for it. We definitely hadn't studied it."

"I wish that he had known more," said Jenny. "It would have been better to know the terrain. The trail was so technical. We didn't realize that. I also didn't know how rural it was. I didn't know where I was. I felt lost, unsure, unfamiliar."

The feeling of isolation extended beyond Southern Appalachia. Weeks before starting the AT, Jenny suffered a miscarriage. Her second. "We both thought I would be pregnant when I was helping Scott. But then I had two miscarriages. After the second one, it was too much. It was just too much stress and too many doctors. I needed a break. I needed an escape.

"The trail was healing for me. It took the miscarriage off the front of my mind. I was finding joy again in simple things, and being together, and being in nature."

In the beginning, the trail was lined with bushes and Bushido. Scott and Jenny were fully in the moment, immersed in the woods, sharing an adventure. They were moving on from two miscarriages, together. Then, after three days—or 155 miles—they entered at Great Smoky Mountains National Park and Scott pulled his right quadricep.

"I was in so much pain," said Scott. "Being a physical therapist, I know what I can run through. And I thought it was over right there."

"Yeah, when he got injured, I thought, well, that's a bust and we're done," said Jenny. "I felt so disappointed."

However, in just a few days, word had spread up and down the trail like an invasive exotic plant that Scott Jurek was trying for the FKT, and when Scott was at his lowest physically, friends and runners, fans and onlookers started showing up at trailheads and hiking or running down the trail to meet him and urge him forward. Despite the injury, he stayed on the trail and hobbled on.

Even once he started to feel better, he didn't run right away. "It's a hiker trail," he said. (More than any of the science that Shawn provided, when Scott said it was a hiker trail, the tortoise in me felt affirmed.)

But there were times when Jenny wished Scott would run. She wished he would run away from the friends, fans, and onlookers who were waiting for Scott and just spend some time with her. "We never had a chance to talk in private because there were always all these people around," she said.

"I didn't know thirty people would be showing up at trailheads," Scott said. "That was *exciting* to me, because people were so inspired. We had our GPS information posted and people just started following us and showing up. I wasn't trying to be social media savvy. I just wanted to document it and include people."

By this time Scott had grown accustomed to sharing his feats of endurance with the general public, but Jenny wasn't used to dealing with all of the attention.

"He had this tracking available and people would come all kitted out to run with him from 5:00 a.m. to the middle of the night. It was still fine, but I did start to get a little bit resentful. He'd be out on the trail. He'd be running in these beautiful places. I'd be in the parking lot talking to all these people. They asked, 'What's he eating? How far is he going?' I just wanted to sleep, do laundry, or read. I didn't want to talk to people. Scott's so used to it, he's so gracious and appreciative. I'm not as extroverted as he is," Jenny said.

On several occasions, runners would come to the trail unannounced to join Scott and then when they were tired or didn't want to run anymore, they asked Jenny to shuttle them back to their cars. Jenny was having enough trouble trying to be Scott's wife, crew, and PR representative. Now she was being asked to be a taxicab, too.

"It's me or the tracker," she yelled. The GPS unit that Scott carried down the trail was held high in her right hand ready to be tossed into the woods. She had just put new batteries in the device, but she wasn't ready to hand it back until she had five minutes alone with Scott.

"The people standing there thought she was kidding. She wasn't kidding," said Scott.

Scott asked the runners standing nearby to go ahead and said he would meet them down the trail. Jenny got five minutes alone with her husband in Massachusetts. That would have to last her until Maine.

June in Vermont was June in Vermont; it was muddy. Next up were the White Mountains of New Hampshire, which reduced Scott to a slow grind. His average pace decreased to less than a mile and a half per hour. It took all his remaining reserves, and very little sleep, less than three hours a night, to make it through Maine on schedule.

But he got to the end. He summited Katahdin and surpassed my FKT by three hours. *That bastard!*

Now I knew exactly how Andrew had felt. It was sad letting go of the record, but at the same time I had a deep appreciation for what Scott and Jenny had accomplished.

"It was the hardest physical thing I've ever done," said Scott. "Running a one-hundred-mile race is different. I'm not saying it's easy. But going day in and day out is a true adventure. The longevity made it the most physically and mentally demanding thing I've done. And just the difficulty of the trail! I've been on a lot of trails, but the AT is different. It's really unique. The hardness, the surface and terrain, plus the history and the trail clubs, then you factor in the eclectic people out there . . . there's no other trail like it."

In a coincidental but poetic detail, the day Scott finished was his wife's birthday. This was her gift. They had set the record as a team. Now they could celebrate by spending time together—alone.

But first, they hiked up to Katahdin with ten of their closest friends and colleagues to capture the record and savor their accomplishment. "The ending was spectacular," said Jenny. "It was a beautiful Sunday afternoon. And the view from Katahdin was amazing. To get there and have the feeling of being done, it was overwhelming."

Once Scott put both his hands on the wooden sign that crowns the summit and bowed his head in reverent exhaustion, it was time to celebrate. But it was the celebration that soon became the focal point of Scott's record.

When he returned to the base of the mountain with Jenny and his team, there were two rangers waiting there for him. They handed him three citations: one for violating the group size limit of twelve people, another for public consumption of alcohol, and a third for littering.

Scott was completely caught off guard and taken aback.

He was offended and upset by the citations, but the full impact of the accusations didn't sink in right away. He had only gotten five hours of sleep over the past three days and he was having a hard time processing everything. His first order of business was to rest and spend time with Jenny on her birthday. He would address the accusations in a few days—with a clearer head.

While Scott was still trying to recover and catch up on sleep, Baxter State Park upgraded his punishment to the twenty-first-century form of public flogging. They put it on Facebook.

"Scott Jurek's recent completion of the Appalachian Trail in the shortest time on record is a remarkable physical accomplishment. With all due respect to Mr. Jurek's ability, Baxter State Park was not the appropriate place for such an event.

". . . Scott Jurek's physical abilities were recognized by corporations engaged in running and outdoor related products. The race vehicle used to support Scott in his run, as well as Scott's headband, clearly displays these corporate sponsors. The sponsors are providing money and equipment to support Scott's run in exchange for advertisement and engagement that they expect will protect or increase their market share and improve their profits.

"Mr. Jurek and the corporate sponsors were careful not to mention in the media coverage that one of the unfortunate outcomes of the celebration party at Baxter Peak at the completion of the event were the three summonses issued to Mr. Jurek by a Baxter State Park Ranger for the drinking of alcoholic beverages in public places, for littering, and for hiking with an oversize group."

If the rangers waiting with citations at the base of the mountain had been a slap in the face, this was a mixed-martial-arts-grade body slam. Scott felt misrepresented, hurt, and confused.

For starters, he did not have a specific sponsor purse or corporate budget for the Appalachian Trail. He and Jenny used their own money to fund the hike. Some of it was income that Scott earned from his sponsors, who put him on retainer and paid him to travel the country to speak and give appearances, but the funds were not earmarked. He could have used the cash to sit on a beach in Cabo.

There were media at the finish, but they traveled there separately from Scott, and most of them had contacted Baxter State Park in advance in an effort to obtain the proper permits. And, yes, one group was a Hollywood production crew who asked if they could fly a helicopter over the mountain, which is akin to asking if you can buzz over the White House or hover with rotating blades above a religious ritual. But Hollywood didn't know any better. And when Baxter said, "No," the film crew obliged.

When it came to his group size, he had started up the mountains and hiked down the mountain with a designated group of twelve people. He had passed other hikers along the way and there had been onlookers who had heard about Scott and waited at the summit to witness his finish, but the size of *his* group never changed.

It was the littering accusation that incensed Scott the most. He had collected nearly four thousand wrappers that summer that had been amassed by himself, his crew, and the people who came to the trail to run and hike with him so that he could recycle them. But according to his ticket, spilled Champagne—even a little, even on rocks, counted as litter.

Scott could not defend the alcohol accusation and didn't intend to try. His friend had handed him a bottle of bubbly goodness. So he shook it up and then took a big foamy sip straight from the bottle before passing it to his crew. "I was tired and it was reflexive," he said. "I wasn't thinking about public consumption laws."

A lawyer from Maine reached out to Scott and offered to help with the citations. "He couldn't believe the way I was being treated and felt I needed representation," said Scott.

The littering citation and the group size accusation were both dropped. Baxter State Park *never* posted that to Facebook. In the end, Scott paid a five-hundred-dollar fine for drinking from a bottle of Champagne on top of Katahdin.

The problems with Scott Jurek and Baxter State Park, the problem with Scott Jurek and fastest known times, and the problem with trying to give an accurate portrayal of him are the same one.

Scott Jurek is a person. He is a dork who wore cutoff blue jeans past their prime, he is a nurturer who loves taking care of his friends and family, and he is an outdoor enthusiast who loves to run, hike, and seek out adventure.

But Scott Jurek is also a brand. He has his own stylized logo composed of his initials, he has corporate sponsors, and he is a noted speaker and author who travels the country to share his message. Sometimes it is hard to differentiate between the two because Scott Jurek's brand and his message are entirely congruent with who he is as an individual.

As a private citizen, Scott has every right to hike the Appalachian Trail—and do it as quickly as he wants. "I did the Appalachian Trail because I wanted to experience it," he said. "There's this perception that I was doing it just because I was a record-hungry trail-running champion, but that's not it. I wanted to see new places. I wanted to meet people on the trail. I would hang out at a shelter for five or ten minutes to talk to thru hikers. It wasn't all about speed. Some people see it as a stunt. It wasn't."

And yet, as a celebrity he sparked a controversy at Baxter State Park that has in part led to a thru hiker permit system at Katahdin. He wasn't the first hiker to drink Champagne, or smoke a stogie, or pot, or crack open a beer on top of Katahdin. But it was his notoriety that gave Baxter the leverage they needed to amend their policies and enforce a cap on AT hikers entering the park.

"I just wished they had called me," said Scott. "They knew we were coming and we could have done something differently. If they wanted to do something productive as far as sending a message to hikers we could have done that. Even, after it happened, I would have been happy to work with them."

Scott Jurek didn't try to bring more attention to FKTs, but in setting the record on the Appalachian Trail he brought a sizable new audience to the sport. He set a standard of publicly declaring intent, tracking progress with GPS, and providing live updates. Not everyone agrees with those practices, but it is hard to deviate from his precedent. Now people are looking for daily updates online and coming to the trailhead to try to catch a glimpse of the next record setter. And the aftermath of his record made it clear that FKT athletes are going to be held to a higher standard than an average hiker or trail runner.

Scott's elevated status changed the world of FKTs—and the policies at Baxter State Park—but his character shows us how to persevere despite negative public perception. He was always gracious to the onlookers who showed up at the trailhead. He showed respect to the record setters who had come before him. He picked up litter and recycled his wrappers. And when he made a mistake, he paid a five-hundred-dollar fine and put it behind him. Scott Jurek shows us how to accept praise and criticism without letting it alter your course.

And that brings us to *Lesson number three: When you try to make everyone else happy you become immobilized. When you accept that you can't, you're able to move forward.* Scott's motives were pure even if his actions weren't. And he demonstrated something on a large stage that every other record setter exhibited in his or her own circle: You can't let public opinion determine the worth of your journey.

Baxter State Park put Scott and his FKT in a negative light. On the other hand, there were a lot of people who never would have considered visiting, hiking, or going for a short run on the Appalachian Trail who were inspired by Scott to take a first step. They were affected in different ways by a journey that was never intended for them.

"I know it strengthened Jenny's and my relationship," said Scott. "It was incredible to work as a team. It was more about the adventure and the trip we had together than the record. It blows me away how physically and mentally empowered I became on the trail. I became empowered not only as an athlete but as an individual."

"It brought us closer together," Jenny added. "And it made us more confident as future parents and reinforced that we did want a family. I got pregnant just two months after the record. And I thought, if we can survive the AT, we can totally survive this."

CHAPTER ELEVEN

The Future of Endurance

"We exist only as long as we persist."

—JPD

Toward the end of my conversation with Scott in Boulder, I asked him how he got across the Kennebec River in Maine, roughly 150 miles from the end of the Appalachian Trail. Every record setter before Scott either took the official canoe shuttle or forded the Kennebec. Fording is the traditional method, but it's also risky. After a hiker drowned while crossing the Kennebec, the ATC started paying someone to ferry hikers and runners across. Since that time, the majority of hikers'—and record setters'— itineraries have been subject to the dictates of the river and the AT shuttle service, which keeps regular hours and has even painted a white blaze on the bottom of the boat to reiterate that it's the official way to cross.

"We took a private canoe across at like, 4:30 or 5:00 that morning. It saved us at least four hours." Scott said.

I choked on the granola I'd ordered. I was speechless. I struggled to process this new information and dislodge the dry oats from my throat.

Scott had broken my record by a little over three hours and he'd just admitted that he'd taken a private boat across the Kennebec River.

"Maybe it was an unwritten thing to take the ATC ferry?" Scott said. "But I got across the river in the traditional way of taking a boat. If I had forded it in my state, it would have been a bad example. It was late in the hike. It wouldn't have been responsible to me or my family.

No one has really come out and said you should do it *this* way. There is a real fine line and sometimes there is going to be a gray area."

Andrew Thompson took the canoe ferry. I forded the river. I thought that Scott should have—would have—followed one of those precedents.

When I shared my findings with Brew, who has the annoying habit of playing the voice of reason, he chalked Scott's approach up to the fact that he didn't really know protocol, either because he came from the running community instead of the hiking one, or because he was from Colorado rather than the East Coast, or because he was just figuring the trail out as he went along.

Regardless of the reason, my conversation with Scott illuminated that when it comes to FKTs, what one person considers off-limits might be fair game to another athlete. I do not think that Scott's taking a private canoe changed the ultimate result that summer. At that point—so close to the end—a person's body is going to do what it needs to do to finish hours or minutes ahead of the previous record. I was reminded that new records and different strategies did not change any part of *my* journey.

When I curled up next to my husband in bed that night, I felt an affirming sense of calm. I reached over to twist off the bedside lamp, then I rested my head deep in the soft down pillow and let out a long, heavy exhalation. The words "it's all good" drifted through my half-waking consciousness, and the ease of ensuing slumber confirmed my response. In a sport with an unwritten rulebook and no physical reward, the primary reward is the *experience*. No one can change that, define it, or take it away from you.

I was drawn to FKT culture by the idea of participating in something underground and disorganized—it's still an amateur sport. There's a kind of kinetic energy to trail records that doesn't exist in other trail pursuits, such as ultramarathons, trail races, and thru hikes.

The word "amateur" comes from the Latin verb *amare*, meaning "to love." That's often how amateur athletics is explained: The individual participates out of personal devotion rather than for financial gain. But true amateurism is elusive.

College athletics are considered amateur pursuits. Yet according to the U.S. Department of Education, Division I college football generated more than $3.4 billion in revenues during the 2013 season. Even youth athletics is evolving into more of a business than a casual after-school activity. As peewee leagues rise in popularity, individuals and club teams are required to participate in tournaments more frequently and pay ever-increasing association fees, both of which generate income for governing bodies.

The increasing demands on wallets and calendars mean more of a strain on athletes and their families, to the point where certain sports are infeasible for children who don't have access to funds, time, and transportation. Scott Jurek fell into this category when his folks couldn't afford football equipment.

Long-distance trails are affordable for everyone. You hop on and hop off the Appalachian Trail and Pacific Crest Trail in most sections without incurring any type of fee. You can picnic at the trailhead and head home or you can go as far as you want as fast as you want.

Fastest known times are unknown to the average sports fan, let alone most Americans. There's no governing body, no cash prize awaiting the victor at the end of the trail. There's not even a free T-shirt.

Trail records seemed to be the essence of what I thought sport should be: a feat in which physical and mental barriers are your greatest adversaries, a pursuit set in a democratic environment that doesn't discriminate on the basis of race, gender, or socioeconomic status, and an activity that is at the mercy of Mother Nature, not some heavy-handed commissioner.

Fastest known times are an ideal—a combination of endurance, integrity, and amateurism. For a record attempt to be successful, the motivation has to be intrinsic. It hurts too bad and asks too much of an individual to be a PR campaign. The greatest reward for an FKT will always be internal. You can't complete a journey of that duration and intensity without gaining a greater sense of self and an appreciation for the people and the environment that surround you. However, as the sport changes, there are fringe benefits.

In August 2016, Karl Meltzer set out from Katahdin to break Scott Jurek's record. Like Scott and David Horton, Karl is an icon in the sport of ultrarunning. He has amassed *thirty-eight* first-place finishes in one-hundred-mile races. That's more than any other runner in history.

For Karl, the AT FKT was the siren that called to him for the better part of a decade. His first attempt was in 2008, but that summer he dealt with a bout of trench foot and came up a week short of Andrew Thompson's 2005 record.

In 2013, Karl went after the mark I set in 2011, but again he fell off pace and bagged it just past the midway point in Virginia. (Karl happens to be an outstanding speed golfer and when he felt the record was out of reach, he traded his trail shoes for cleats and hit the links. In a feat even more obscure than an FKT, he once set a world record for playing 230 holes of golf in twelve hours.)

Three years later he returned, hungrier than ever, this time gunning for Scott's newly cemented time. With more than thirty-five hundred miles of Appalachian Trail experience, "Speed Goat," as he's known in the trail running world, knew exactly what—and who—he was up against.

For more than fifteen years Scott and Karl have competed against each other on the ultra scene, and the Appalachian Trail was the ultimate backdrop and proving ground for their rivalry. Despite the fact that they were on the trail different summers, they were effectively competing in their longest and perhaps final race against each other.

For five weeks, Karl nipped at Scott's heels. With fewer than five hundred miles to go, Scott flew from Boulder to crew and run with his longtime friend and competitor over the final ten days of the journey. There are many accounts of past record setters helping rivals with prehike logistics and spending time with them on the trail. Warren did this for me on both of my record attempts. But I'd never heard of a current record holder offering so much assistance to the person trying to break his mark. Scott's display was a testament to sportsmanship, to friendship, and to him as a person.

When Karl reached Springer Mountain in Georgia, he had surpassed Scott's record by a little less than ten hours and had become the first athlete to move the record under forty-six days. In an amusing twist, he broke his vegan friend's record by eating junk food, swilling beer, and downing energy drinks.

Karl's caffeine intake provided a physical and financial boost. His AT attempt had been more or less bankrolled by Red Bull, the energy drink company that backs adrenaline-pumping skateboarders, surfers, mountain bikers, and the like.

When an interviewer asked Karl afterward how much he'd spent on the record attempt, he said it was north of $100,000. When I heard that figure, my jaw dropped. Most PCT and AT thru hikers budget a couple bucks a mile, depending on how many hotels they stay at and where they food shop. Not factoring in gear and transportation to and from trailheads, a thru hike or record attempt routinely runs $4,000 to $6,000.

This was a lifelong pursuit of Karl's. He was all in, his sponsors were fully behind him and, like Scott, Karl had earned the right to chase his dream after spending decades at the pinnacle of his sport. These guys took chances where others didn't, and those risks paid off. But here's the catch—and one of the things I love the most about FKTs. The gal with a shoestring budget is still going to be able to compete with that guy cashing sponsorship checks. You can buy a better support vehicle, you can buy a bigger audience, but you can't buy endurance.

One reason sponsorship money has become available for athletic pursuits that take place in the middle of nowhere is the advent of GPS tracking devices. In the past, FKTs were solitary endeavors, but technology has made it possible to follow athletes on websites and social media, which makes record setting in the wild an engaging endeavor and a viable business opportunity.

Besides giving instant access to fans, tracking devices can also serve as a means of verifying record attempts—or in some cases casting serious doubt on them.

Heather Anderson was one of the first record setters to track her progress by GPS. When I asked her if modern FKT athletes should use GPS as a standard practice, she quipped, "Only if they want people to believe them." But Heather suffered an unexpected backlash when the live updates she released on social media resulted in well-wishers tracking her down on the trail, bringing encouragement and food. Those bonus calories Heather received caused some to question the purity of her "self-supported" hike. Thru hikers often accept "trail magic" and record setters do the same, but the assistance should be serendipitous. The fact that these "trail angels" had singled Heather out made some people question whether it qualified as unacceptable assistance on a self-supported hike.

When Heather set the record on the Appalachian Trail, she took the opposite approach and did not offer live information, so as to avoid controversy and unwanted encounters with well-wishers. She still posted updates online, but they were delayed by several days. Then, more or less out of the blue, she arrived at Springer Mountain, having shaved a remarkable four days off the previous record. Eventually she released her data to the hiking community to substantiate her claim, but folks criticized her lack of transparency. Heather tried to do the right thing, two different ways, and received flak both times.

When Scott Jurek posted on Facebook that he would be serving up live updates on his AT record attempt, I thought it was a huge logistical mistake. He did have a lot of local hikers come out to help him down the trail and provide moral support, but he also lost buckets of time glad-handing and taking pictures with fans at trailheads. When I asked him whether all the people showing up was more a help or a hindrance, he said it was probably a wash.

The biggest consequence of sending live updates was that it made life very hard for Jenny, who was waiting with the throngs of followers for Scott to come out of the woods. Beyond the emotional strain of being constantly surrounded by well-intentioned runners, Scott also worried that he might be putting his wife at risk. "We were on all these rural back roads and I just worried that the wrong type of person might try to find Jenny while I was on the trail," he said.

GPS isn't foolproof and it never will be. Units run out of batteries. If they fall to the ground—which is a distinct possibility on rugged terrain—they can break. And that's not to mention more nefarious scenarios. As Andrew Thompson points out, "If someone wants to cheat, all he has to do is send a crew member down the trail with his GPS while he shuttles the support vehicle around to the next road crossing and catches some extra shut-eye."

Technology is a tool, and it is becoming standard practice to include GPS tracking on an FKT attempt, but unless there is a chip implanted in an athlete's arm, trail records will continue to depend on the record setter's honesty.

I wondered what past record holders thought about establishing some sort of governing body and creating "best practices" to substantiate trail records, and when I asked them, the responses I heard were mixed. Even if we standardize the rules, we can't standardize the trail. Each hike is unique and the conditions on the trail never repeat themselves. That's something the budding FKT community has been grappling with.

In 2016, a Belgian man claimed the FKT on the Pacific Crest Trail but freely admitted that he took shorter reroutes and at one point skipped an entire section due to fire closure. In each case he was just doing what was suggested by the path's governing association. He was following official trail detours and using common sense rather than risk heavy fines by traversing dangerous terrain covered in conflagrations. Some people view his mark as the new FKT record. Others write it off completely or consider it a record with caveats.

Calamities aside, with so many ways to differentiate attempts, FKTs run the risk of being overrun with subtle distinctions. Should a northbound record be any different from a southbound? Should there be separate male and female categories, even though women have proved they can compete with and beat men? What about a professional category for sponsored athletes and an amateur one for weekend warriors? The categories could break down ad infinitum.

These questions should serve as a reminder that the completion of a long-distance trail is always a remarkable accomplishment of endurance. Many of the most impressive feats on the Appalachian and Pacific Crest trails have absolutely nothing to do with speed. To know that someone can walk two thousand plus miles in less than two months is no less mind-blowing than the fact that *three* separate five-year-olds have walked the Appalachian Trail. The Appalachian Trail Conservancy and Pacific Crest Trail archives hold stories from the first legally blind individuals to hike each path, as well as men and women who have thru hiked a dozen times or more. There have been yo-yos and winter traverses and hikers with notable physical and mental differences—including amputees, diabetics, people with Down syndrome, autism, and cystic fibrosis, men and women dealing with PTSD and severe depression. All were willing to crawl even when they couldn't take another step.

When it comes to FKTs there are more record attempts, more controversial claims, more sponsored athletes on the trail, and more women in the mix. But trail records are still a small part of a much larger landscape.

Brew is often baffled that I don't follow the record attempts with a closer, more critical eye. He and several of our trail friends try to track the major record attempts and make sure that each athlete is holding him- or herself to a high standard of transparency and integrity. He is much more active than I am in exposing poor form and untruths within the world of FKTs, especially on the Appalachian Trail.

He says that it matters because of how hard we worked to set the record. Brew also knows the effort that our friends and peers put into their FKT accomplishments. He doesn't want anyone to disrespect the mark that we set, the record that Warren held and that David Horton surpassed, the FKT that Andrew Thompson went after four times, and the title that Scott took from us and that Karl Meltzer then claimed. Brew is right. What we did, and what these other athletes have accomplished, does matter and should be protected from falsities and slander.

But the farther removed I am from our trail record, the less interested I am in the minutiae of the sport and the more focused I am on what binds us together as athletes, outdoor recreationalists, and human beings.

Now more than ever, we need to keep this stuff in perspective. Our national trails face unprecedented challenges. Usage is skyrocketing at the same time that funding is being cut, water rights are being litigated, and companies are threatening to build pipelines and power lines across trails or to mine or strip timber in proximity to trails.

Those of us who love wilderness are all on the same team. The biggest issues facing FKTs are real and important. They are the same issues threatening to affect birders, fisherman, foragers, and mountain bikers. If we don't join forces on major issues, there will be no reason to debate the minor ones.

Every record setter I talked with suggested that he or she was lured or called or drawn to the trail by something deep inside his or her being. There is an invisible force that pulls individuals of varying interests and pursuits *back* into the wild. Our existence has been tied to the natural environment since the beginning of humanity. Yet in an effort to protect ourselves from the elements we have walled ourselves off, not just from storms, but also from sunsets. We have protected ourselves from unsavory individuals, as well as friends and neighbors. And we have found a way to stay healthy by sanitizing our society and synthesizing our food and drugs. This is not natural, or safe, or healthy.

The problems to be addressed are not our biped pace. There is a small difference between traveling two miles per hour, four miles per hour, and six miles per hour. There is a big difference between man-powered locomotion and driving seventy miles per hour down the interstate. It is the speed and distance of our commutes and the breakneck pace of life that are the cause for concern, not FKTs.

In our overregulated society—which searches desperately and constantly for a sense of control—trail records are a messy, realistic reminder of how liberating life can really be when you stop comparing yourself to other people and focus on exploring your own potential. The essence of endurance will never be defined by rules and categories; it will be distinguished by the stories of the unique individuals who blaze the trail. And the value of trail records comes from the tangible life takeaways exemplified by the men and women who travel the thin dirt path in search of their capabilities and identities as creatures of endurance.

It is all too easy to forget how resilient we can be physically and emotionally. All of my close friends and family members are dealing with problems that challenge them and call into question their ability to persevere. The effects of divorce, infertility, or depression are faced daily by many of my loved ones. Personally, I question my ability to run a business, be a devout wife, mother, and friend, stay physically active, and feed some small piece of my soul apart from those commitments. And that's when things are going well. Throw in financial upheaval, a friend dealing with cancer, or a family tragedy and I question whether I have the strength to continue moving forward with effectiveness or compassion. My FKT experience and my role models within the sport embolden me to stick it out, and I believe that these specific examples of endurance can cast a net of empowerment far beyond the reach of a niche trail community.

When I spent time with Warren I was reminded of the dangers that come with complacency. It is easy to follow the path that is laid before us even if it isn't a good course or the right direction. Warren made me realize how important it is to ask questions of your society, your community, and yourself. We have to assess our abilities and our surroundings before we can chart our course.

Endurance can be exposed through tragedy and life's greatest challenges, but it can also be revealed and used through conscious questioning. Our resilience is proved in trying circumstances and exhibited by accepting a challenge. Choosing to tackle difficult situations will help us better navigate the ones that are forced on us.

The fact that Warren is in his late sixties, with a Santa Claus physique, helps us recognize that endurance isn't just for athletes in their prime. Warren's legacy is not found in setting a trail record in his twenties, but in hiking the entire Appalachian Trail nearly twenty times and helping other people successfully complete the path. Warren set a mark that was surpassed by a runner, but he has left a mark on the trail—and on me—that extends in perpetuity.

David Horton helped me to understand that you don't have to overcome your insecurities to achieve greatness and that dealing with self-consciousness is not a one-time struggle, but a lifelong battle. He taught me that you don't have to get rid of the pain to move forward. The hurt we experience in life might not ever fully go away; it could ebb and flow for an eternity. You can make progress and appreciate the times when life isn't as much of a struggle. And you can pray, and cry, and wrestle through the rest.

Horton and I agree that purpose is essential to forward motion. We find this motivation in our faith; not everyone does. Some, like Andrew Thompson, find their drive in escaping organized religion. Others say that they don't need a transcendent purpose to press forward. Endurance is for both the religious and the irreverent, but I still think it doesn't hurt to have a higher cause. When you're uncertain whether you have the power to face the obstacles ahead, it helps to have faith that something bigger than your ability will meet you in times of trouble.

To this day, Horton is so worried about losing that he can't appreciate or understand how much he has done well. But that doesn't stop him from trying. The man who lost his firstborn at the hospital, almost lost his leg to a freight accident, and lost his ability to run due to a knee injury is still moving. As he approaches the end of his seventh decade, he is still married, still teaching, still directing ultra races, and in 2017 he biked across the United States in thirty-two days, averaging 133 miles per day. He wrecked his bike and fractured his shoulder, but he still finished. Despite the pitfalls, he has persisted.

The trail records set by Warren Doyle and David Horton are milestones in the history and formation of FKTs. Their marks have been surpassed, but they should not be forgotten. These men take different approaches to endurance and life, but they have both made great strides and along the way they have also become friends. The trail may be a literal line in the sand, but it is not a dividing line. Instead it invites men from both sides to come to the middle and walk together.

The current FKTs will fall and change hands. However, I am more concerned about recording the history of trail records than trying to keep track of every new attempt, because if we can appreciate where the sport has been, it helps us approach the future as a better-informed and unified force. The same holds true for our country and our quality of life.

Do not let the news channels inform your opinion of other people. The democratic ideals of America are represented by long trails and libraries and liberty for all, not fear mongering and stereotyping. Whenever an issue is portrayed as us versus them, no one will win. Go outside, take a walk with someone who is different from you. You might not agree with him or her, but you will learn to respect that person. We must protect and appreciate our common ground.

Our heritage is connected to the land—and movement. The story of humanity is one of constant forward motion. Admit to yourself that you are a mover. You have evolved from a *Homo erectus* species that has spent thousands of years tracking prey, following herds, searching for reliable food sources and safety, walking to holy sites, and caravanning to markets. Ignite that spark of activity that lies dormant in your being and let it grow. When you start to move, it might hurt and feel uncomfortable, but ultimately you will discover a feeling that suggests you are accomplishing a purpose that your body was designed to achieve.

Don't be afraid of failure. Endurance is failure, after failure, after failure. Scott Williamson shows us that fulfillment isn't found in accolades or public recognition, but in the ability to get back up after falling short of a goal. He dropped out of school and walked away from a home of emotional abuse and a community of crime to find his own path. You are defined by your upbringing and life's tragedies only if you allow yourself to be a victim of them. You don't have to accomplish great things because of your past or in an effort to escape it, but you can accomplish great things in spite of it.

Scott Williamson illustrates that a lack of formal education does not determine your intelligence. Books are sustenance for the self-taught, and the lessons of experiential education are far more valuable than memorizing facts. There is a language to surviving—and surviving outdoors. Don't forget to include this in your studies.

After coming within a quarter of an inch of being paralyzed or killed, Scott Williamson tried to complete the first PCT yo-yo and failed five times. He also lost his best friend to suicide and lost contact with his daughter. But, today, he has two successful yo-yos to his name and three FKTs. He has a wife who loves him, understands him, and protects him. And he has hope that he can continue to improve his PCT records and his relationships.

I have a sense that things are going to work out for Scott Williamson, because he is going to keep trying to make things better for the rest of his life. Endurance is consistently telling yourself that it is going to be okay regardless of the immediate circumstances and past events. It is okay to fall short, it is okay to let people down, it is okay to hurt and suffer, it is okay to stop when you can't go any farther. But don't give up on yourself, your goals, or the people around you.

Being relentless doesn't have to be a grind, it can be fun loving and politically incorrect. There is liberation in defying the status quo that can bring out the rebel in us all. Andrew Thompson teaches us how to enjoy the struggle and shows us how relational endurance can be. Going the long haul is more bearable when you're able to laugh at setbacks, laugh at yourself, and tackle the obstacles ahead with a zeal for life.

We might all go farther if we end each day with a cold beer and a good friend. Andrew, along with every other record setter, demonstrates how crucial teamwork is in helping an individual accomplish something extraordinary. Whether it is a spouse, relative, or best friend—like J.B.—every record setter has received strength and encouragement from a loved one. If that person is going after a supported record, then he or she has also received calories, companionship, and an occasional kick in the ass. You have to have someone great in your corner if you want to accomplish something outstanding. And when the tables turn, you'd damn well better be in that person's corner. Support goes both ways.

If we recognize our own need for forgiveness, it becomes easier to extend that favor to those around us. Andrew helps us understand that you have to forgive the people who are closest to you if you want to keep them in your life. He also shows us how to accept our flaws and our strengths and not try to hide either with false humility.

Most of us could benefit from sharing in Andrew's confidence—and he might be well served to off-load a little of it, but I'd rather have too much than not enough. Believing in yourself and your own ability is crucial to performance. When you know you're going the distance, being self-assured allows you to continue forward with less anxiety and doubt. It gives you more freedom to enjoy the journey. Having confidence will help you obtain the result you've envisioned—even if it takes a couple of tries—because your mind has already informed your body of the outcome.

My experience on the trail helped me realize that I don't have to go through life shelving my thoughts, ambitions, and accomplishments in a women's category. At this time, no female has surpassed my mark on the Appalachian Trail, yet I don't profess to have the female FKT. I competed with the men, I beat the men, and I want my mark to remain in the overall category—even if I'm lower on the list. I am tired of having asterisks placed next to my name because of my gender. I proved that I belong and I'm not going to let anyone put me in a different division.

I also don't want the next woman who comes along to compete with me. I want her to pit herself against Scott and Karl or whoever holds the FKT title at that time. I figure if a woman is going to take down my time, then she might as well take down the guys', too.

Removing the labels of gender does not strip you of your femininity, but helps you to excel beyond a category.

As soon as I walked off Springer Mountain, I realized that the value of setting an FKT is not found in recognition, or held in cherished memories, it is manifested in its application to everyday life.

After Scott Jurek broke my record, I was called multiple times by different newspaper writers and magazine editors to get a quote concerning his accomplishment. It made me feel like a commentator, and I didn't want to be a commentator; I wanted to be a participant.

I confronted the fact that I wasn't challenging myself or taking risks. I was busy caring for my family and company, but I wasn't caring for my soul. I wasn't asking myself what exciting and terrifying opportunities I could test myself with and I wasn't putting myself in a position where I could fail. I needed to be more like Warren; I needed to ask myself, What can I strive for now?

I didn't want to try for another trail record, but I did want to set *the* record straight. The reporters who interviewed me were never able to fully portray trail records or the athletes who participated in the sport because they didn't understand it. I wanted to write the real story. But I didn't have the credentials or contacts to make that happen. I knew what I wanted to do, but I was mired in self-doubt.

When a reporter from the *New York Times* called me to talk about Scott Jurek, I decided not to let the conversation end without making my own pitch. A few weeks later I was emailing writing samples and an article outline to the sports editor at the *Times*. Thank you, Scott Jurek, for that contact. And thank you, David Horton, for teaching me how to put myself out there despite my self-doubt.

I worked for two years on my book, and I was pregnant or nursing nearly the entire time, not to mention other obstacles that reared their ugly heads. There were the gender-specific demands placed on my body and there were the sweet rewards that come with mothering a newborn baby, but I was not going to let the reality and responsibilities of my sex affect my ability to deliver a manuscript. If anything, I convinced myself that the creative aspects of bringing life into the world were going to enhance my ability to cultivate something amazing in my writing.

As I worked on this project in the confines of my basement office, I followed Heather Anderson's adventures online and via text messages. Receiving updates from her always made me smile. It made me grateful for what I have and what I was doing, but it made me proud to have a friend like Heather who was redefining possibility and fulfillment.

Endurance can be pecking away at your keyboard late at night with a baby sleeping next to you—and frequently waking up. It can also be setting a record on the Arizona Trail, or hiking the remote Oregon Desert Trail with your boyfriend, or traveling around the country in a small truck to bag high points. Following a traditional path works for most individuals, but if you ever find yourself feeling misplaced in our modern American culture there are other options. Hiking long trails and existing on very little income is a viable alternative. Traveling the world to pursue adventure and explore unmarked terrain can provide more satisfaction than living out the American Dream. Choosing not to have children will allow you to nurture something besides the next generation. These decisions are not socially irresponsible; on the contrary these choices offer a way to minimize the resources that you need and that you use. If you feel as if you don't fit in where you are, you are not stuck. Feeling stuck is no excuse for staying where you are. Life is hard; struggle is guaranteed, but you can exercise your right to choose where and how to struggle. Learn to move forward with imperfections.

When Brew and I are in the car and we pass a runner or walker on the sidewalk, it is natural for my husband to make comments about how fast or slow they're going and what their stride looks like. My rule of thumb is that you never judge someone else's pace or form, because you don't know how far they've come and what they're still planning to do.

We all have our long trails, and most of them do not include much hiking or running. Outside the forest, our paths take the form of higher education, climbing out of debt, navigating a career, staying married, undergoing divorce, surviving tragedy, and coping with illness. It behooves us to not come to quick conclusions about other people's paths and instead approach each individual with encouragement and compassion. We might be on different trails, but we are all midjourney.

Hikers love acronyms. We constantly write them in trail registers and spell them out loud. One of my favorites is AYCE, which stands for All—You—Can—Eat. But perhaps, the most common and philosophical is HYOH, Hike—Your—Own—Hike. I went into this project hoping to find the similarities between endurance athletes, and what I discovered is that there are very few commonalities. I will say that those of us who attempt to harness the power of endurance through FKTs are not prone to groupthink: The past, conventional wisdom, the rules, or even our own limits cannot dissuade us from rising to the challenge. We learn to accept pain, embrace adversity, and come through the other side not just stronger but better than before. But we all do it differently.

There is no formula for perseverance. It's not rooted in diet or physical training. It's not based on a person's background or bank account, and it can't be compartmentalized into purely physical characteristics. At the end of the day, it must be attributed to a single commonality: being alive. Our mere existence qualifies us as creatures of endurance. Some of us are more conscious about it than others, but each morning we wake up, breathe in life, accept the challenge, and try to go a little farther than the day before.

Humans have the capability to change course. We are not driven by evolutionary impulses to the same degree as other members of the animal kingdom. We can assess, rationalize, and approach each action with critical thinking. We can train our habits and control our actions. This should be empowering; we are not a product of our environment, but we are still subject to it and accountable for it. Our ability to make choices that affect our direction can also affect the people and the world around us. We are able to create and destroy in a manner that no other species can.

People won't work to protect something if they don't value it; and we typically don't value something unless we experience it. Before I started hiking, conservation was not high on my list of priorities. Now I think about it daily. My main motive in caring for the environment is not to protect and preserve the earth for the sake of the earth, but to do it for the sake of people. I've come to the conclusion that Mother Nature wins. We can't outmuscle her, control her, or outlast her. She is the ultimate endurance athlete. Our course of increased consumption and disregard for the environment will be far more devastating for humans than for our planet. I don't know what it will take to shift our global priorities and I shudder at what that wake-up call will be, but I am confident that as humans we are able to change our direction and effect positive change. Moreover, I believe we will. We have too much at stake not to. At the end of the day we are all survivalists.

Our tendency toward perseverance is demonstrated globally but felt most deeply at an individual level. Whether you choose a difficult challenge to unveil your capabilities or are forced into a situation that seems like more than you can bear, rest assured that the struggle is not in vain. Our journey forward is about more than survival. Every obstacle that we overcome allows us to acquire strength, gain wisdom, and internalize gratitude. The sacrifice demanded is never wasted; instead it provides an education. It teaches us about other people, it teaches us about the world around us, but more than anything, it teaches us that we are more resilient and powerful than we ever dared dream.

We all have incredible gifts, and very few of them will be

manifested in laying down miles on a long dirt trail. For each individual, the greatest feat of endurance comes in uncovering his or her talents and applying them in a way that makes his or her life—and world—a more beautiful, compassionate, and daring adventure. There are amazing inventions, innovations, acts of love and service that happen each and every moment. And there are countless accomplishments and contributions that outweigh the importance of FKTs.

On the longest journeys and the longest records, differences disappear. Gender, age, diet, and ideology lose their distinction—and we are stripped down to creatures of struggle and imperfection and resilience; we are stripped down to that which binds us together. The greater the distance, the easier it is to see that we are all just human. And as humans we need to work together to continue forward. Endurance isn't a human trait; it is *the* human trait. We exist only as long as we persist. And there is confounding hope and limitless possibility in our ability to rise up, change direction, and take one more step.

ACKNOWLEDGMENTS

As much as this is a book about endurance it is also a tale of teamwork and support. I am indebted and grateful to everyone who has been a part of this project. From its inception to its completion and as it continues to find its legs and audience, this project has felt significant. In the manner in which our team has been able to convey authentic stories with enthusiasm and respect, and in the way this book transcends a sport and touches on important modern issues, it feels like we have—together—accomplished something great.

Thank you to my literary agent, Kirsten Neuhaus. Kirsten, you helped me turn an article—and a dream—into a compelling book proposal. You have also made me feel heard throughout the entire process. I appreciate your strong communication and I admire your tenacity.

When I met Laura Tisdel at Viking, I knew that she was the right editor for this project, and I am so grateful that we were able to work together. Laura, you are a creature of endurance! Thank you for giving me and everyone around you your best self. Your feedback and vision have turned this manuscript into a book that goes beyond the hiking and running communities and encourages individuals in every walk of life.

To everyone else at Viking, I appreciate your backing and I am in awe of your talent. Thank you to Brianna Harden for a beautiful cover; thank you to Brianna Linden for the strong publicity push; and thank you to Amy Sun for not letting anything fall through the cracks.

I will also always be filled with gratitude for my relationship with my first publisher, Eric Kampmann. He believed that I could both hike and write and he gave me the chance to prove myself as an author. Eric, thank you for setting me down this path and walking with me for so much of the way.

The pictures on the book jacket were taken by a friend on one of my favorite stretches of the Appalachian Trail. They were also taken at 6:30 a.m. with clouds, wind, and rain rolling through—and my young children sleeping nearby in a tent. Chris Galloway, thank you for taking a chance, braving the weather, and capturing something beautiful.

I wrote this book while trying to keep my babies and my business growing healthy and strong. I couldn't have accomplished that without Christine Martens's excellent management of Blue Ridge Hiking Company, Haley Blevins's love and care for my children, and Lauren Fortuna's constant friendship and willingness to do whatever she could to help me meet my deadlines.

This book would not carry the same weight and significance if it were solely the reflections and opinions of one person. I wanted to tell the stories of my friends and colleagues because I knew that their accomplishments on the trail had not been told with the depth, history, and context that they deserved. I was hopeful that these individuals would trust me with their experiences, but I was humbled when they invited me into their homes for days at a time and shared not their greatest accomplishments but their greatest struggles and regrets. I am filled with admiration and fondness for Warren Doyle, David Horton, Scott Williamson, Andrew Thompson, Heather Anderson, and Scott Jurek. These individuals have served as my personal role models and I know they will inspire countless other men and women.

I also want to acknowledge the accomplishment of Joe McConaughy. Joe, you're fast . . . but not fast enough! I wish I could have included you in this book. A forty-five-day self-supported traverse of the Appalachian Trail is phenomenal—and a significant step in the evolution of fastest known times.

I called on several sources and friends to make this book informative and compelling. Thank you to Brian King, Peter Bakwin, and Ward and Cathy Leonard for your insights and edits. And I owe a special debt of gratitude to Daniel Czech and Shawn Bearden for being my sounding boards and expert sources on the science and psychology of endurance.

Finally, I am fortunate to share my life and love with a man who has supported my dreams and become a part of them. Brew Davis, thank you for being my partner in endurance.

BIBLIOGRAPHY

These books were helpful for my research and were an inspiration for *The Pursuit of Endurance*:

Hare, James R. *Hiking the Appalachian Trail.* Vol. 1, Rodale Press, 1975.

Horton, David, and Rebekah Trittipoe, *A Quest for Adventure: David Horton's Conquest of the Appalachian Trail and the Trans-America Footrace.* Lynchburg, Virginia: Warwick House Publishing, 1997.

Jurek, Scott, and Steve Friedman. *Eat and Run: My Unlikely Journey to Ultramarathon Greatness.* New York: Houghton Mifflin Harcourt, 2013.

McDougall, Christopher. *Born to Run: A Hidden Tribe, Superathletes, and the Greatest Race the World Has Never Seen.* New York: Alfred Knopf, 2009.

Dr. Seuss. *Horton Hatches the Egg.* New York: Random House, 2004.

Dr. Seuss. *Horton Hears a Who.* New York: Random House, 1954.

Shaffer, Earl V. *Walking with Spring: The First Thru-Hike of the Appalachian Trail.* Appalachian Trail Conference, 1983.

Shostak, Marjorie. *Nisa: the Life and Words of a !Kung Woman,* Cambridge, Massachusetts: Harvard University Press, 2000.

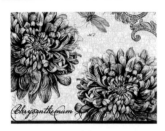

Chrysanthemum

In memory of
ELIZABETH "SAM" WILKERSON